Examining Complementary Medicine

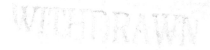

Examining Complementary Medicine

'THE SCEPTICAL HOLIST'

Edited by

Andrew Vickers
Research Council for Complementary Medicine

Stanley Thornes (Publishers) Ltd

© 1998 Stanley Thornes (Publishers) Ltd

First published in 1998 by:
Stanley Thornes (Publishers) Ltd
Ellenborough House
Wellington Street
CHELTENHAM
GL50 1YW
United Kingdom

98 99 00 01 02 / 10 9 8 7 6 5 4 3 2 1

A catalogue record for this book is available from the British Library

ISBN 0-7487-3314-0

Typeset by WestKey Ltd, Falmouth, Cornwall.
Printed and bound in Great Britain by
TJ International, Padstow, Cornwall.

Contents

List of contributors

Saul Berkovitz is a doctor at the Royal London Homoeopathic Hospital, Great Ormond Street, London WC1N 3HR, UK. (*Chapter 2*)

Stephen Birch is an acupuncture clinician, instructor and researcher at the Anglo-Dutch Institute for Oriental Medicine, Kennemerloon 162 1972 ES IJmuiden, Netherlands. (*Chapter 3*)

Anthony Campbell is a teacher and practitioner of homoeopathy and acupuncture. Correspondence should be addressed to: 8 Oak Way, London N14 5NN. (*Chapter 11*)

David M. Eisenberg is a physician. He directs the Center for Alternative Medicine Research, Beth Israel Deaconess Medical Center, 330 Brookline Avenue, LW-600, Boston MA 02215, USA; and is Assistant Professor of Medicine at Harvard Medical School. (*Chapter 1*)

Peter Fisher is Director of Research at the Royal London Homoeopathic Hospital, Great Ormond Street, London WC1N 3HR, UK. (*Chapter 5*)

Bob Fordham is a homoeopath and teacher at the School of Homoeopathic Medicine and the Sheffield School of Homoeopathy. Correspondence should be addressed to: 14 Greenfield Place, Ryton-on-Tyne, Tyne & Wear, NE40 3LY. (*Chapter 7*)

Maria Hondras is a chiropractor and researcher at the Western States Chiropractic College in Portland, Oregon, USA. (*Chapter 14*)

Ted J. Kaptchuk is a practitioner of Chinese medicine and associate director of the Center for Alternative Medicine Research, Beth Israel Deaconess Medical Center, 330 Brookline Avenue, LW-600, Boston, MA 02215, USA. (*Chapter 1*)

George Lewith is a doctor who practises a number of complementary therapies. He leads a complementary medicine research unit at the University of Southampton. Correspondence should be addressed to: University Medicine, Level D, Centre Block, Southampton General Hospital, Tremona Road, Southampton SO16 6YD, UK. (*Chapter 13*)

David Peters is a doctor who practises a number of complementary therapies and teaches at the Centre for Community Care and Primary Health, University of Westminster, 115 New Cavendish Street, London W1M 8JS, UK. (*Chapter 10*)

Ursula Sharma is Professor in Sociology at the University of Derby. She has specialised in sociological study of complementary medicine. Correspondence should be addressed to: 60A Derby Road, Fallowfield, Manchester M14 6US, UK. (*Chapter 12*)

Caroline Stevensen is a holistic health consultant and practitioner with a background in social sciences and nursing. Correspondence should be addressed to: 19a Kildare Gardens, London W2 5JS, UK. (*Chapter 6*)

Jeremy Swayne is a medical homoeopath and a member of the Faculty of Homoeopathy. Correspondence should be addressed to: Greys, Ditcheat, Shepton Mallet, Somerset BA4 6RB, UK. (*Chapter 4*)

Stephen Tyreman is an osteopath who co-ordinates postgraduate studies at the British School of Osteopathy, London. Correspondence should be addressed to: Melville Lodge, 102 West Lodge, Lincoln LN1 1JZ, UK. (*Chapter 9*)

Andrew Vickers is a researcher at the Research Council for Complementary Medicine, 60 Great Ormond Street, London WC1N 3JF, UK. (*Introduction*)

Clive Wood, Department of Biological Anthropology at the University of Oxford and Centre for Community Care and Primary Health, University of Westminster, is a former Council member of the British Holistic Medical Association. Correspondence should be addressed to: 30 Elmthorpe Road, Wolvercote, Oxford OX2 8PA, UK. (*Chapter 8*)

Preface

The idea for this collection of essays came from a conversation about a book called *The Sceptical Feminist* (Radcliffe Richards, 1982). I was told that this criticises many common feminist beliefs and arguments. What seemed most important about the book was that its author, Janet Radcliffe Richards, is a well known feminist. In other words, the book provides criticism from within.

What had happened in feminism, Radcliffe Richards argues, was that the debate had become polarised between proponents and opponents. Criticism became seen as a weapon: feminists 'criticised' the organisation of society and the behaviour of men; conservatives 'criticised' feminists. What had become lost was the use of criticism as a tool to examine and develop one's own beliefs.

Radcliffe Richards' general point was that feminists needed to be more self-critical. As she puts it, her book is, in part, a battle 'against a good deal of common feminist dogma and practice'. The intended result is for feminism to have 'firmer foundations, less vulnerability to attack. . . . more general acceptability'. Radcliffe Richards' purpose in criticising feminism was not destructive; rather, she sought to strengthen it and to help bring about its goal, which she saw as the creation of a just society.

Talking about *The Sceptical Feminist* brought to mind numerous parallels with complementary medicine: the polarised debate; the lack of self-criticism; the reformist zeal coupled to insufficiently explored 'dogma and practice'. And so I thought of 'The Sceptical Holist': a collection of essays offering critiques of complementary medicine written by people working within it.

Over four years later, I finally compiled the papers for *Examining Complementary Medicine: The Sceptical Holist*. I view the project both as a failure and as a success. It is a failure in the sense that my original vision – a large number of closely argued papers examining specific topics in complementary medicine – has not been fulfilled. But, in retrospect, perhaps this vision mistook means for ends. What I have observed in the last three years is an almost revolutionary change in the ability and willingness of the complementary medical professions to engage in critical self-appraisal. All of those writing in this book have contributed to that change. I have little doubt that our association with 'The Sceptical Holist' has developed our own critical abilities and helped us to articulate critical ideas more fluently. In this sense, the project has already achieved a degree of success.

That said, the criterion by which this book will be judged is whether, in the long term, it contributes to the development of critical discourse in complementary medicine, whether it forges the link between academic rigour and practical reform – the tempering of creative ideas with discriminating judgment – which is such a powerful force for social progress.

Andrew Vickers 1998

REFERENCE

Radcliffe Richards, J. (1982) *The Sceptical Feminist*, Penguin, Harmondsworth.

INTRODUCTION

Criticism, scepticism and complementary medicine

Andrew Vickers

I seem to have had to be on the defensive against your continual criticism;
I wonder if you are basically an unhappy man to have to spend your
energies in decrying other people's efforts rather than adopting a more
positive, cooperative, friendly and helpful approach.

Part of a letter to the author from a complementary practitioner.

INTRODUCTION

This paper will make two very simple points. Firstly, criticism is a good thing.
Secondly, there is not enough of it about. The overall argument is that
practitioners of complementary medicine have interpreted criticism and scepticism in a manner that has not served their own best interests: 'criticism' has
been taken to mean denigration rather than analysis; 'scepticism' has been
understood in the negative sense of distrust and disbelief, rather than in the
positive sense of a cautious attitude towards accepted truths.

I will start by examining the evidence that critical self-analysis has been rare
in complementary medicine. I will then discuss possible reasons including, on
the one hand, the social, educational and professional structure of complementary medicine, and on the other, the appropriation of the language of
criticism by those politically opposed to unconventional medical techniques.
The adverse effects of the lack of self-criticism in complementary medicine will
be considered in brief before concluding with a general analysis of why
criticism and scepticism are of benefit in health care.

As an early proviso, I wish to state that it is difficult to make generalisations about a field as broad and heterogeneous as complementary medicine. It is likely that much of what I say will be more appropriate to certain professional groups than to others. That said, I do believe that it is worth coming to some general conclusions about criticism, scepticism and complementary medicine.

CRITICAL SELF-ANALYSIS IS RARE IN COMPLEMENTARY MEDICINE

Turn to just about any book on complementary medicine and you will usually be hard pressed to find even a single statement that criticises any theoretical or practical aspect of the therapy concerned. Most books are characterised by long lists of claims, stated baldly as matters of fact. As an example, I have just opened a book selected at random from my bookshelves. The *A–Z of Natural Therapies*, written by Judy Jacka, an Australian practitioner and teacher of natural therapies, seems a fairly standard complementary medicine text. Large numbers of statements are made about the cause and treatment of disease, for example, 'homoeopathic doses [are useful] for removing plaque and balancing the cholesterol metabolism' (Jacka 1994, p. 82). At no point does the author provide a critical analysis of these statements. There is no examination of whether the claims are either valid or useful. Furthermore, the author generally neither tells us why she is making a particular claim (is it based on personal experience, the opinions of an expert or perhaps the results of scientific research?) nor gives us any reason why we should believe in it: often no argument or evidence is presented for or against. As a result, the reader cannot make any form of critical evaluation. You either believe or you don't.

The *A–Z of Natural Therapies* is not an isolated or unusual case. Elsewhere (Vickers, 1996), I have examined aromatherapy textbooks and found enormous numbers of unsubstantiated claims, e.g. 'Lavender and Neroli . . . will help to reduce scars.' (Davis, 1988, p. 95.) I decided to write to a number of leading authors and ask them on what basis they had made the claims presented in their books. Most failed to reply; one author said he had nothing to add to his published writings and another sent a letter stating that she refused to cooperate. One initially claimed that his book was based upon scientific research but declined to continue any correspondence when challenged on this point. If we are not told the basis upon which aromatherapy claims are made, we have no method of evaluating them. Again, there is no opportunity for critical debate: you either believe or you don't.

Some authors of complementary medicine books do reference the scientific literature to justify knowledge claims. But such referencing often has an unusual feature: only positive evidence is ever used. Only when there is research available that lends support, however indirectly, to an author's prior beliefs, will the scientific literature be cited. As it happens, commercial organisations are selling research data to complementary practitioners for precisely this purpose. For example, the cover sheet for data provided by the Natural Therapies Database explicitly links research to self-justification: 'I know only too well of this need to justify my work and teaching with . . . research. Proof is now at your fingertips!'

References to negative evidence are almost entirely absent from books by complementary practitioners: certainly Jacka (1994) does not provide any. In my reading of the literature, I have not come across any instances where an author has said something along the lines that 'we used to believe or do X; then research evidence emerged that X was either wrong or not in the best interests of patients and we have now stopped doing or thinking X.' On the rare occasions when authors report research results that do not support current practices or beliefs, it is the research which is normally criticised. Existing practice and belief become the standard by which evidence is measured rather than the other way round. An alternative strategy has been simply to quote the research and ignore its result. Lawless (1994, p. 97), for example, supports her suggestion that lavender is of benefit for perineal healing after childbirth by referencing a study that found no difference between treatment and placebo (Dale, 1994). The use of research as a prop to support prior beliefs precludes it playing a useful role in a critical and evaluative discourse.

But we do not have to go to the literature to find obstacles to critical evaluation in complementary medicine. Certain professional groups have actually enshrined their opposition to critical evaluation in codes of practice. Perhaps the most well known example is the *Practice Guidelines for Straight Chiropractic* (World Chiropractic Alliance, 1993). These describe the individual practitioner's clinical assessment as 'inviolable' and his or her judgement as 'the final authority.' A profession will clearly not be able to engage in critical self-evaluation if individuals are given the right to hold as sacrosanct their own personal opinion. Even more explicit is the Code of Ethics of the International Society of Professional Aromatherapists (1990), a leading UK aromatherapy organisation. Paragraph 3.4 states 'Members must present a united front to the public and should not imply criticism of colleagues either in writing or before clients or the general public.'

In sum, critical self-evaluation has hitherto been rare in complementary medicine. Statements made by authors in the literature are presented in a way that precludes critical evaluation and it is not unknown for organisations to proscribe critical activity.

THE STRUCTURE OF COMPLEMENTARY MEDICINE IS AN OBSTACLE TO CRITICAL DISCOURSE

Education

Complementary medicine is largely private medicine. Generally speaking, the organisations that teach complementary therapy do not receive public funds;

the regulations governing practitioners are not determined by public representatives and therapy is not reimbursed by state insurance or national health systems. There have been several important implications for criticism in complementary medicine. At its most basic level, the lack of state funding for complementary therapy education puts a premium on rapid completion of clinical training. Where funding is sparse, students will want to qualify and start practice as soon as possible, so that they can pay back debts incurred for fees and living expenses. Though there are notable exceptions, and though the situation appears to be changing (Research Council for Complementary Medicine, 1995), colleges of complementary medicine tend to offer the teaching of a trade rather than higher education. What is taught is diagnosis and treatment, only rarely is there an opportunity for the development of critical, reflective and analytical skills.

The development of training institutions in the private sector has also had the effect of distancing complementary therapy education from the university setting. The effect of this has been profound because the university is the cradle of critical thinking, of analysis, of healthy scepticism towards accepted wisdom. It is where new ideas are tested and developed, where, arguably, the most significant scientific, social, philosophical and humanities research is undertaken. Though there may have been benefits from developing outside the university system, complementary medicine has been cut off from a fertile source of creative and critical thinking and lost access to the human, technical and financial resources that are vital for good quality research.

Complementary medicine, alternative culture?

It is, no doubt, false to say that those who practise complementary medicine necessarily adopt beliefs and behaviours associated with 'alternative' culture. To date no author has provided evidence that complementary practitioners tend, for example, to squat empty houses, eat unusual foods, smoke cigarettes made from plants other than tobacco or wear unconventional clothing.

That said, there is a pervading belief that complementary medicine constitutes a general criticism of conventional behaviours and beliefs. Proponents of complementary medicine do not typically present their therapies as only another useful addition to those techniques already available to alleviate human distress. Instead, they often use their therapy as a springboard for a wide-ranging attack on conventional approaches to health, nutrition, science, epistemology and life in general. It is not just that a particular complementary therapy can be helpful and should be used more often, it is also made out that modern living is unhealthy and unnatural and, moreover, that biomedicine is fundamentally flawed because it ignores the placebo effect and relies on the out-dated Newtonian clockwork model of the universe (Micozzi, 1996). Again the aromatherapy literature provides a useful example:

Computer screens . . . are responsible for many illnesses . . . Drugs . . . lower the immune system, other factors include: antibiotics; stress; VDUs; excess sugar; stimulants such as coffee . . . television.

Tisserand (1990, pp. 7–71).

This embedding of complementary medicine within a broader social and cultural critique has two effects on the development of critical discourse. Firstly, criticism becomes something that is directed solely outwards. Criticism is not something for self-evaluation, it is what is used to attack others. Secondly, because one form of critical evaluation, scientific research, is seen as embedded in a socio-cultural *status quo*, it becomes the subject of bitter hostility. For example, Scheid (1993) claims that 'the scientific re-evaluation of traditional systems of medicine . . . amounts to acts of epistemological violence.' Though at least some of the claims made about conventional research techniques do hold – just as many of the broader cultural critiques found in the literature are valid – one of their effects has been to hinder critical self-evaluation in complementary therapy. The randomised trial, attacked so vociferously by many complementary practitioners, is, after all, a useful method of evaluating whether the care provided by health professionals is actually of benefit to patients. It is the means by which, for example, a number of dangerous and ineffective surgical treatments have been rejected (Turner *et al.*, 1994).

Professional structure

Complementary medicine is largely practised by individuals working from their own homes or private clinics. Even where practitioners do work together – at 'natural health centres' and the like – they do not generally cooperate in the care of individual patients. Furthermore, many complementary therapies are not regulated by a single governing body. Not only does there tend to be a number of separate regulatory organisations for each therapy but these are frequently at odds with one another. Often, different schools founded by different individuals promoting different methods of practice and a different philosophy of care found their own regulatory bodies, which register graduates from only a single training institution.

The professionally diffuse nature of many complementary therapies has had a negative effect on critical self-evaluation. If practitioners tend to work alone, they are less likely to be subject to the views of those with a different perspective. It also fosters a spirit of therapeutic individualism, given ultimate expression in straight chiropractic's injunction against 'violating' the 'final authority' of the individual practitioner. Furthermore, by working alone, practitioners tend to miss group interaction and discussion. In a typical hospital, groups of doctors, nurses, researchers and other health professionals meet weekly to discuss case histories, clinical problems and research projects.

It is possible to see interprofessional critical discourse in action at lunch time in the seminar room. This is something that generally could not be said of the private practitioner, working solo in the community.

The break-up of different schools of thought in complementary medicine into opposing factions has also stifled the development of critical thinking. Not only do criticism and scepticism become directed outwards, at those who do not practise a therapy 'properly', but practitioners become surrounded by like-minded individuals. Under no pressure to challenge their beliefs, practitioners are able to work in cosy isolation, untroubled by the difficult and sometimes painful process of critical self-evaluation.

Tradition

As Coward (1989) points out, virtually no complementary therapy advertises itself as being new. As a particularly crude example, a recent brochure for transcutaneous electric nerve stimulation – an unequivocally hi-tech therapy – claims that its origins are to be found with the ancient Egyptians, who, allegedly, used electric eels for medicinal purposes. Similarly, a leading aromatherapy author claims that 'the history of the application of essential . . . oils to the human body must be almost as old as history itself' (Arnould-Taylor, 1992, p. 6). This is a remarkable claim given that most essential oils are obtained by distillation, a process that was not invented until the ninth or tenth century. The most extreme case of reliance on tradition is found in acupuncture, where most modern textbooks make copious reference to classic Chinese texts, many of which are over a thousand years old.

This reverence for tradition has a predictable effect on critical thinking. If tradition makes right, if the ultimate authority is the texts of centuries old books, if to find knowledge we look only backwards, then the progressive impulse of evaluative discourse becomes irrelevant. Criticism and scepticism have no place in systems of thought that are determined solely by tradition.

A similar point could be made about the role of the 'founding figures' in complementary medicine. Hahnemann, Still, Palmer, Alexander, Feldenkrais, Bowen, Trager, Rolf, Heller, Rosen, Schussler, Bach, Voll, Reich, Fitzgerald, Gerson: the list of founding figures whose names still pervade the literature is almost endless. What is of particular interest is that the stated origin of many therapies is the same – a single unusual event experienced by a single individual: Alexander loses his voice; Palmer cures a deaf man; Ignatz von Peczely notices a stripe on the iris of an owl with a broken leg. This mythologising of the therapy's birth as *revealed* to a founding figure stifles critical evaluation by making closeness to a static historical ideal the sole criterion by which ideas and practices are judged. It would be inconceivable to argue that, say, Bach was right about the properties of most of his flower essences but that he mixed up hornbeam and white chestnut. The Bach flower remedies are perceived to be a complete, timeless and unchanging system, divinely revealed to Edward

Bach in the Oxfordshire countryside of pre-war Britain. Critical evaluation becomes irrelevant, tradition is all.

Defensiveness against attacks

Practitioners of unconventional medical therapies have commonly been subject to verbal assaults, professional censure and even legal proceedings. Doctors have been struck off for practising complementary therapies or even for mere professional association with alternative practitioners (see, for example, the case of F.W. Axham (Inglis, 1980, p. 69)). Similarly, the careers of some academics (such as Jacques Benveniste) have been ruined for investigating complementary medicine. Complementary practitioners themselves have been harassed by regulatory authorities, forced into exile (Hoxsey being a well known example) or incarcerated. Perhaps the most notorious case is that of Wilhelm Reich, an important figure in the history of psychoanalysis, who was prosecuted in the 1950s for activities associated with his 'orgone box.' Reich's books and papers were burnt and he was sent to prison, where he died (Inglis, 1980, p. 109).

Verbal abuse of the practices, practitioners and patients of complementary medicine is a less overt form of attack, but nonetheless results in damage to the cause of criticism. For example, Petr Skrabanek, a well known 'critic' of complementary medicine, described those who use it as 'bleeding prey for the sharks roving the seas of medical ignorance' (Skrabanek, 1988).

Though persecution and abuse of this sort is thankfully no longer common, practitioners of complementary medicine remain understandably defensive. The idea of criticism has come to be interpreted in entirely negative terms. Criticism is equated with political attack; critics are those who wish to denigrate, dismantle and destroy. The creative and progressive aspects of criticism – those of analysis and reflection – become obscured by the more pressing requirement for self-preservation.

THOSE WHO ARE POLITICALLY OPPOSED TO COMPLEMENTARY MEDICINE HAVE APPROPRIATED THE LANGUAGE OF CRITICISM

As far as I am aware, there is only one book on complementary medicine which currently includes the phrase 'critical analysis' on its jacket. *Examining Holistic Medicine* (Stalker and Glymour, 1989) is said to 'offer a comprehensive collection of essays . . . that critically analyzes the theory, methods and practices of holistic medicine.' Unfortunately, the essays are all written by political opponents of complementary medicine, those who have a uniformly negative opinion and who wish to have their views enforced by legal and professional censure. One editor has stated that he would still have zero belief in homoeopathy even if 'a hundred randomized, double-blind clinical trials' were conducted and all had positive results (Stalker 1995). Despite such extreme prejudice, he feels justified in recommending his book to 'licensing boards; those who construct licensing examinations; politicians, legislators and jurists who must decide what legal role to give holistic medical practices, federal funding agencies [and] insurance companies' (Stalker and Glymour, 1989, p. 9). Interestingly, this quote appears on the very first page of text. *Examining Holistic Medicine* is not a book that 'critically analyzes' complementary medicine with a view to constructively improving the services offered to patients, it is a work of advocacy, an attempt to malign and ridicule as a prelude to political control.

In the opening essay of the book, holistic medicine (used as an approximate synonym to complementary medicine) is described as 'nonsense offered by cranks and quacks and failed pedants who share an attachment to magic and an animosity toward reason' (p. 26). Each of the following papers involves a focused, destructive attack on a specific topic. E. S. Crelin's paper on chiropractic (Crelin, 1989) is a typical example. Crelin introduces chiropractic as an 'unscientific cult' (p. 197). Setting out to 'convince the public', he decides to 'attack the chiropractors directly with the facts', an activity he equates with trying to 'debate the Russians at the United Nations.' With no qualms about taking the rhetorical high ground ('I was really a low-paid basic scientist with no axe to grind but the truth'), Crelin worries not only about the capacity of chiropractic to 'maim or kill' but also about its effects on society as a whole ('millions of dollars of taxpayers' money have filled the pockets of chiropractors') and raises the issue of fraud (patients of chiropractors are described as 'unsuspecting people who are willing to let the quacks fleece them of their money'). Crelin ends his essay with the words 'innocent children', proof enough of his adversarial stance and emotive tone.

Examining Holistic Medicine is a classic example of the appropriation of critical language by those politically opposed to complementary medicine. Critical analysis, the express purpose of the book as described on its jacket, becomes what an opponent of something does when he or she sets out to attack it. Being critical is equivalent to being against.

A further illustration of how criticism has been equated with advocacy and adversarial rhetoric is provided by an issue of *The Skeptic*, an American publication dedicated to promoting 'science, skepticism and critical thinking'. Issue number 1 of volume 3 is dedicated to 'Pseudomedicine' and includes papers on specific therapies such as homoeopathy and therapeutic touch as well as general articles on 'Prime time quackery' and 'Alternatives to scientific health care'. The cover shows a rather stern-looking nurse with rays emanating from her hands, a picture apparently designed to be insulting to practitioners of therapeutic touch.

The paper on homoeopathy is 'a position statement by the National Council Against Health Fraud'. It includes recommendations that the US

Federal Trade Commission 'review advertising of homeopathic products . . . for false and misleading claims' and 'take action against advertisements . . . used to indoctrinate salespeople, who will in turn deceive consumers'. State legislators are encouraged to 'abolish state licensing boards for homeopathy' and to prohibit 'homeopathy in the scope of practice of any health care provider.' Medical licensing boards are asked to 'discipline homeopathic practitioners' and to 'prosecute nonphysicians engaging in homeopathy.'

In short, opponents of complementary medicine have appropriated the language of criticism for political ends. The result is that 'critical thinking' entails an adversarial 'position statement' recommending draconian state control, prohibition and prosecution. 'Science' and 'skepticism' come to involve the automatic assumption that 'alternatives to scientific health care' are necessarily quackery and pseudomedicine.

THE LACK OF CRITICISM IN COMPLEMENTARY MEDICINE HAS LED TO IT BECOMING OVERBURDENED WITH UNDER-EXPLORED CONCEPTS AND PRACTICES

The adversarial stance of *Examining Holistic Medicine* is particularly disappointing because a number of telling points are mixed in among the abusive language. A few examples will be given here, not in the name of point scoring against complementary medicine, but as a demonstration that critical discourse raises interesting issues and debates.

Stalker and Glymour's opening paper points out that at least some of what is claimed in holistic medicine is merely a restatement of obvious features of any good system of medical care. Examples include awareness of the links between mind and body and an understanding of the multifactorial aetiology of many conditions: 'such banalities are often true and no doubt sometimes ignored, with disastrous consequences, but they scarcely amount to a distinctive conception of medicine'.

In the paper on nursing, Williams, (1989) attacks the idea that 'holistic nursing' is really anything new. Using a similar argument to Stalker and Glymour, Williams criticises holists for appropriating the language of good medicine, examining, in particular, the claim that holistic nursing is somehow more 'caring' than traditional practices. She also points out that proponents of holistic nursing have often based arguments on inadequate data – such as poorly documented case histories – and attacks the belief that holistic nursing must necessarily involve unconventional techniques such as therapeutic touch or reflexology.

One of the strongest essays in *Examining Holistic Medicine* is that of Austen Clark (1989), who tackles the issue of psychosomatic disease. Clark examines the claim – often made by self-described holistic physicians such as Kenneth Pelletier – that illness is all or nearly all psychosomatic. Clearly important in any such claim is the definition of 'psychosomatic'. Clark argues that proponents of holistic medicine do not have a coherent theory of how mind and body interrelate. He points out that holistic practitioners, while criticising conventional medicine for its dualistic conception of mind and body, appear to rely heavily on dualism when they claim, for example, that negative emotions can cause physical disease.

A similar point is made by Wikler (1989). Practitioners of complementary medicine often discuss 'personal responsibility' for health. Yet 'responsibility' has numerous different meanings, at least some of which are connected to guilt and liability (for example, 'he was responsible for the loss of the ship'). Moreover, the ability of individuals to control ('take responsibility for') their health is affected by complex interactions between a large number of factors: genetics, socio-economic status and environment being just three of the most obvious. Complementary practitioners seem to pay scant regard to this complexity when they claim, for example, 'we are responsible and are accountable for our feelings, thoughts, beliefs, morality, ethics, behavior and actions in relation to others' (Flynn, 1980, p. 26).

Stalker and Glymour's own paper (1989b) focuses on the claim that recent advances in quantum physics refute the assumptions of conventional medicine and support those of complementary practitioners. This claim ignores the fact that quantum effects are extremely small. Moreover, it conflates the use of a theory because it brings about successful results with the use of a theory because it is believed to be objectively true; after all, satellites are still flown by Newtonian physics. Stalker and Glymour challenge proponents of 'quantum healing' to produce a single quantum calculation which contradicts any biomedical finding. They point out that although some conventional understandings – such as that of the separateness of observer and observed, or that of cause – do break down in certain quantum phenomena, they remain useful approximations. The assumptions and methods of biomedicine should not be discarded wholesale just because they do not hold in certain extreme, non-biological situations.

Even Crelin (1989), whose text is weighed down with abusive and adversarial comments, raises a number of important issues. He points out that chiropractic is based on the theory of 'subluxations' of vertebrae, and that these subluxations have never been shown to exist. In fact there is good evidence that they do not. Crelin's paper is also of value in its discussion of the useless and possibly dangerous machines used by some chiropractors, the unusual nature of many chiropractic claims and the basic anatomical errors found on some chiropractic anatomical charts.

The global and esoteric criticisms found in *Examining Holistic Medicine* may be complemented by a look at how complementary therapies are used in practice. Even the most preliminary analysis of complementary practice highlights the profound difficulties that have arisen from a lack of critical discourse. Take as an example a woman suffering from premenstrual syndrome who visits a male homoeopath. A number of different questions might be asked. In which circumstances should the homoeopath treat her and in which refer her on somewhere else? Which of the various homoeopathic materia medica should he use? In what way should he ask questions in order to reach a diagnosis? What potency and dose of remedy should be given? Should he prescribe only one or a combination of different remedies? When should the woman return for evaluation? At what point should the remedies be changed? What other advice would be appropriate? Should the woman avoid coffee and camphor, which are said to negate the effects of homoeopathy? What should she be told about her overall prognosis?

It should be apparent that without reliable answers to these questions homoeopaths will not be able to offer the best possible service to their patients. But, as it happens, probably no such answers are known: it is doubtful whether any aspect of homoeopathic practice has been subject to sufficient critical evaluation. That homoeopaths nevertheless often do feel confident in answering questions such as those above – presumably on the basis of their professional opinion or that of their teachers – is evidence that practitioners of complementary medicine have largely failed to appreciate the importance of criticism and scepticism.

IS CRITICISM REALLY A GOOD THING?

As stated in the introduction, this paper aims to make two points: that criticism is a good thing and that there is not enough of it about. Thus far, I have provided evidence for the latter point and explained both its origin and consequences. But what of the former claim? Is criticism really a good thing?

Debates about epistemology – how to find out about things – are essentially metaphysical. It is difficult to provide evidence for a methodology because the evidence will typically be provided in the terms of that methodology. I could argue that criticism was a good thing by comparing those professions that have and have not incorporated critical discourse, but that would itself be a critical argument. I could also point out that it is wise to be sceptical about our beliefs, because throughout history people have often been in error, but again that would be to use a sceptical argument to argue for scepticism. In short, we can never know for sure whether complementary therapies would be better off remaining as static historical traditions or would be improved by the development of criticism. It can and has been argued that in analysis – a word synonymous with 'dissecting' or 'breaking down' – it is possible to miss what is fundamental. Does a critical evaluation of a meal make it any more delicious? Can an art critic make a sculpture more beautiful? Is complementary medicine any different?

There is, though, what I believe to be a final and convincing argument for criticism and scepticism in health care. It relates to what health care is all about: the individual in distress. Criticism is how we can aim to ensure that healing modalities are conducted so that they benefit the patient. Without criticism and scepticism, what takes priority are the views of the practitioner, handed from teacher to apprentice like a sacred flame. If I criticise a therapy, I do so on behalf of those who might benefit from it. If I refuse to do so, I put the therapy before the patient.

In sum, it is time to rescue criticism for complementary medicine. Its current role – forgotten or even forbidden by complementary practitioners; used as a weapon by political opponents – is a sterile one. By reclaiming critical and sceptical thinking, and becoming 'Sceptical Holists', practitioners of complementary medicine can ensure that they offer their best to themselves, their profession and especially their patients.

REFERENCES

Arnould-Taylor, W.E. (1992) *A Textbook of Holistic Aromatherapy*, Stanley Thornes, Cheltenham.

Clark, A. (1989) Psychological causation and the concept of psychosomatic disease, in *Examining Holistic Medicine* (eds D. Stalker and C. Glymour), Prometheus Books, Buffalo, NY.

Coward, R. (1989) *The Whole Truth*, Faber & Faber, London.

Crelin, E.S. (1989) Chiropractic, in *Examining Holistic Medicine* (eds D. Stalker and C. Glymour), Prometheus Books, Buffalo, NY.

Dale, A. and Cornwell, S. (1994) The role of lavender oil in relieving perineal discomfort following childbirth: a blind, randomised clinical trial. *Journal of Advanced Nursing*, **19**, 89–96.

Davis, P. (1988) *Aromatherapy: An A–Z*, C.W. Daniel, Saffron Walden, UK.

Flynn, P. (1980) *Holistic Health: The Art and Science of Care*. Robert J. Brady Co., Bowie, MD, p. 26.

Inglis, B. (1980) *Natural Medicine*, Fontana, Glasgow.

International Society of Professional Aromatherapists (1990) *Code of Ethics*. International Society of Professional Aromatherapists, Hinckley, Leicester.

Jacka, J. (1994) *A–Z of Natural Therapies*, Lothian Books, Melbourne.

Lawless, J. (1994) *Lavender Oil*. Thorsons, London.

Micozzi, M.S. (1996) Characteristics of complementary and alternative medicine, in *Fundamentals of Complementary and Alternative Medicine* (ed. M.S. Micozzi), Churchill Livingstone, London.

Research Council for Complementary Medicine (1995) Report of the working party on research education in schools and colleges of complementary medicine. Research Council for Complementary Medicine, London.

Scheid, V. (1993) Orientalism revisited. *European Journal of Oriental Medicine*, **1**(2), 23–33.

Skrabanek, P. (1988) Paranormal health claims. *Experientia*, **44**(4), 303–9.

Stalker, D. and Glymour, C. (eds) (1989a) *Examining Holistic Medicine*, Prometheus Books, Buffalo, NY.

Stalker, D. and Glymour, C. (1989b) Quantum medicine, in *Examining Holistic Medicine* (eds D. Stalker and C. Glymour), Prometheus Books, Buffalo, NY.

Stalker, D. (1995) Evidence and alternative medicine. *Mount Sinai Journal of Medicine*, **62**(2), 132–43.

Tisserand, M. (1990) *Aromatherapy for Women*, Thorsons, Wellingborough.

Turner, J.A., Deyo, R.A., Loeser, J.D., *et al.* (1994) The importance of placebo effects in pain treatment and research. *Journal of the American Medical Association*, **271**(20), 1609–14.

Vickers, A.J. (1996) *Massage and Aromatherapy: A Guide for Health Professionals*, Chapman & Hall, London.

Wikler, D. (1989) Holistic medicine: concepts of personal responsibility for health, in *Examining Holistic Medicine* (eds D. Stalker and C. Glymour), Prometheus Books, Buffalo, NY.

Williams, S.M. (1989) Holistic nursing, in: *Examining Holistic Medicine* (eds D. Stalker and C. Glymour), Prometheus Books, Buffalo, NY.

World Chiropractic Alliance (1993) *Practice Guidelines for Straight Chiropractic*, World Chiropractic Alliance, Chandler, AZ.

PART ONE

History

This section examines how history can be used both to promote and to prevent critical discourse in complementary medicine. Ted Kaptchuk and David Eisenberg's essay on the history of granola (a health food product similar to muesli) demonstrates that in order to understand contemporary ideas, one must uncover their social and cultural origins. Ideas about health and treatment do not arrive fully formed out of thin air: they are created by particular people at particular times and are informed by the beliefs and prejudices of their creators and developers. The alternative health food movement can be characterised by the manner in which diet has been used to promote particular moral and political beliefs. Saul Berkovitz's essay is based on a comparison between his own academic research on the life of Edward Bach, inventor of the Bach Flower Remedies, and the histories of Bach given by his followers. He points out that the 'official' story of Bach's life is at best an oversimplified historical account and at worst an inaccurate one. He then goes on to examine the function of the 'myth of Bach' as that of stifling critical appraisal of Bach's work and of protecting commercial interests.

Health food or granola: its truth and consequences

1

Ted J. Kaptchuk and David M. Eisenberg

INTRODUCTION

Alternative dietary lifestyles are important forms of alternative healing practices. The themes of 'Nature', vegetarianism and social/spiritual regeneration provide a persuasively attractive and integrative vision for many people. The paper looks at the history of alternative dietary practices in order to examine the meanings and morality embedded in their approach to healing.

FOOD AND DIETARY LIFE STYLES AS MEDICINE

In the pursuit of health, many people routinely treat cancer with a regime centred on brown rice (US Congress, Office of Technology Assessment, 1990; Bowman et al., 1984; Cassileth et al., 1984), seek relief from arthritis with a variety of other diet therapies (Brown et al., 1980; Kronenfeld and Warner, 1982), confront chronic fatigue with an array of nutritional supplements (Herbert, 1980; Reed et al., 1989) and promote well-being with 'organically' grown food (Jukes, 1977; White, 1972). According to the often cited *New England Journal of Medicine* survey of alternative medicine in the United States, food-related unconventional medical practices constitute one of the leading forms of alternative health care (Eisenberg et al., 1993). These food-related practices, which form a 'complex and specialized nutritional health healing system' (Hongladeron, 1976), are used by millions of people at a total of billions of US dollars (Harris & Associates, 1987; Cowart, 1988). In some cases, the practices of alternative dietary reform overlap with those of biomedicine: eating foods low in fat or high in fibre would be examples. This essay, however, concerns alternative dietary beliefs and practices that do not conform with the standards of the biomedical community (Gevitz, 1988). An attempt will be made to uncover the network of medicine, meaning and morality embedded in this maze of food practices.

Dietary reform movements confront an observer with a broad assortment of practices. Central to many such practices is vegetarianism in various forms and degrees (e.g. with or without dairy products and/or eggs) (Dyer, 1982). Preparation can range from none, in which case all food is eaten raw (including the possibility of fruitarianism) (Bloomfield, 1983; Ehret, 1953; Kulvinskas, 1981), to all food cooked, in which case the diet centres around grain (Anon., 1989; Frances, 1976). Foods can have special symbolic significance bearing 'overtones of magic' (Gifft and Washbon, 1972), wheat sprouts can have 'growth force' (Kandel and Pelto, 1980), vitamins and large dosages of nutritional supplements give an extra boost of energy or protection from illness (Fried, 1984; Herbert and Barrett, 1981), and carrot, spinach or lettuce juice possess special rejuvenating properties. Exaggerated claims of power can extend to a wide assortment of foods, including wheat germ, yoghurt, black strap molasses, brewer's yeast, grape juice, lemons, seed sprouts and apple-cider vinegar (Todhunter, 1973). Especially potent products such as shark cartilage (considered by some to have immune properties, because sharks are thought not to get cancer) are sometimes acceptable, even if one subscribes to vegetarianism (Lane and Comac, 1992). Likewise, different 'schools' of diet therapy have different food avoidances: macrobiotics will not eat tomatoes and potatoes (Anon., 1989), and Hay diet followers do not mix carbohydrates and protein (Todhunter, 1973). The perception that sugar and white flour are a diabolic threat to health and well-being is shared by most approaches (Mogadam, 1990).

Typically, leaders of this sprawling and eclectic movement are lay people who claim to be able to understand the laws of nutritional science, medicine and nature better than the scientists of the age (Green, 1986; Herbert and Barrett, 1981). Paradoxically, however, scientific findings are selectively applied to argue for the system used (Dubisch, 1981). Among those who follow one practice or another, some join partially in pursuit of particular or general improvements in their health; others engage in an all encompassing sense of participation in an alternative lifestyle and world view. In some cases, diets and lifestyle are not so much ends in themselves, but are pursued in order to enhance more esoteric social, political or spiritual goals consistent with a religious–cultural movement. For example, it is argued that one can pursue the practice of yoga, meditation, world peace or being a psychic healer more easily if one is a vegetarian (Kandel and Pelto, 1980). Both 'unitary users', who subscribe to a particular system or follow a particularly charismatic leader and 'general users', who try a variety of approaches, participate in the movement (New and Priest, 1967). As a whole, dietary lifestyles and health food represent one of the most informal and free-flowing of alternative medicine practices. 'The movement exists primarily as a set of principles and practices rather than an organization' (Dubisch, 1980).

A loose network of charismatic travelling lecturers, commercial stores and restaurants, residential programmes and retreats, manufacturers and distributors, alternative health care providers, exercise teachers and media – not to mention various books, journals advertisements and classes – maintain and inform a vague cohesiveness and allow for different layers of commitment and participation (Kandel and Pelto, 1980, p. 341).

THE CORE BELIEFS AND HISTORICAL CONTINUITY OF THE HEALTH FOOD MOVEMENT

To an outsider, the polymorphous and even contradictory forms of health food, available in smorgasbord fashion, makes this entire healing approach seem chaotic and even bizarre. Until recently much of the biomedical literature has labelled these movements as 'fads' or 'cults' or 'quackery', with the implication that they are transitory phenomena peripheral to mainstream culture. In fact, these movements are a persistent and enduring part of the health care scene with a history of almost 200 years which is parallel to and allied with more clearly delineated alternative therapies such as homoeopathy, Mind Cure or chiropractic (Fuller, 1989; Whorton, 1988, 1989). Underlying this history a consistency and coherence emerge.

The modern natural or health food store with its wooden panelling, sacks of coarse grain, shelves of heavy wholegrain breads, bottles of vitamins, books on organic food and vegetable juices and bins of herbal preparations is a continuation of the first Graham provision store (after Sylvester Graham, see below), which the American Physiological Society opened in 1837 in downtown Boston. This store sold coarse wholegrain products made from produce grown according to 'physiological principles' (the nineteenth-century equivalent of 'organic') on 'virgin unvitiated' soil – soil that had not been subjected to the 'overstimulation' of manure (Hoff and Fulton, 1973). This type of store was reincarnated under more modern nomenclature when a Kneipp water-cure supply centre began to style itself a 'health food store' in New York City at the turn of the nineteenth century (Cody, 1985). The British had previously in the third quarter of the nineteenth century been using the term 'health depot' (Nissenbaum, 1980). Various features of the health food movement have undergone a similar process, emerging as new avatars of their former selves over the course of the past two centuries.

Despite myriad practices and theories, and countless new leaders and spokespersons, three core beliefs and sensibilities underlie the health reform movement both at the present time and throughout its history. The first is Nature; the second vegetarianism; and the third is the belief that dietary reform is a crucial step in the general rehabilitation and regeneration of society. Nature, for most of these dietary systems, represents the 'ultimate standard of legitimacy' and the iconographic repository of virtue (Twigg, 1979). The emergence of the Nature theme in dietary reforms coincides with the replacement of the household economy with industrial manufacturing and the market economy in the early decades of the nineteenth century. Nissenbaum points out that as late as 1800, 85% of America's manufactured goods were produced in the household, and the bulk of these goods was consumed either by the family that made them or by a neighbouring household in the same community. By the 1830s, this figure has been reduced dramatically. For many people, within a single generation, the household had ceased to be the basic unit of production (Gutman, 1973; Nissenbaum, 1980).

The decline of an intimate relationship with the natural environment, on the one hand, and the rise of industrialisation and the market economy, on the other, converged to allow the development of a nostalgic romantic view of nature and what Oliver Wendell Homes once called 'the nature-trusting heresy' (Warner, 1978). Nature is not 'red in tooth and claw' but beneficent, innocent and wholesome (Coward, 1989). The positive valuation of low-level technology and the demonification of unnatural 'chemical,' 'artificial,' 'toxic' and 'technological' interventions have their original formulation here. Positive images of self-sufficiency, individual responsibility and self-help are also rooted in the idealisation of household economics.

Vegetarianism, in various diverse forms, is a second core belief of dietary healing. The vegetarianism of the last 200 years markedly differs from what was earlier called Pythagoreanism (Taylor, 1965). This earlier vegetarianism entailed a subduing of the flesh in order to facilitate spiritual development. The body was considered a handicap to the spirit. In contrast, the new vegetarians and health reformers of the last two centuries have glorified physical wellness. Unlike earlier ascetic traditions, the new vegetarianism of the health food movement lauds embodiment. 'A spiritual body . . . is being stressed, not a disembodied spirit.' (Twigg, 1979, p. 22). The new vegetarianism and health reform movement sees the body as perfectible; it 'offers a this-worldly form of salvation in terms of the body. It is a purity movement, but one that operates fully through the concept of the pure body' (Twigg, 1979, p. 22). Nature is perfect, embodiment can be glorious, and right eating allows for the mutual commingling and interpenetration of the sacred and human. Not only desirable and possible, perfection of the body is viewed as a precondition to spiritual or religious edification.

Thirdly, alternative dietary reform has generally been connected to other kinds of reform movements with the understanding that the effects of diet are so broad as to have larger moral, social or religious implications (Beckford, 1984; Harrison, 1987). While an ordinary supermarket may have a bulletin board posting community events, the notices in a health food store more routinely concern issues of ecology, feminism, political reform, animal rights, Tibetan freedom, world peace, racism, nuclear destruction, poverty, famine and a great assortment of new religions (McGuire, 1988). Nor is this new. Earlier food movements were also allied with alternative health, politics and spiritualism. For example, the 1855 meeting of the American Vegetarian Society, which took place at the leading New York City hydropathic healing centre, counted among its participants the suffragette Susan B. Anthony, the clothing reformer Amelia Bloomer and the anti-slavery advocate and spiritualist fellow traveller Horace Greeley (Nissenbaum, 1980, p. 150).

GRANOLA: A HISTORICAL CASE STUDY OF MEDICINE, MORALITY AND MEANING

Underlying radical dietary reform and its themes of Nature, vegetarianism and reform lies a complex metaphor of virtue and meaning. This dimension of health food practices becomes particularly apparent when one views the phenomena over time. A good example of this, and one that serves as a useful case study, is the history of granola, a paradigmatic American natural food, created by toasting a combination of various grains (especially oats), fruits and nuts (Anderson, 1978). The European equivalent of granola is muesli, the uncooked 'perfect food' created by the Swiss physician Max Bircher-Benner, who died in 1939 (Bircher-Benner, 1959). The story begins with the two earliest advocates of health reform in the United States: Sylvester Graham (1795–1851), of Graham cracker fame, and William Alcott (1798–1859), cousin of transcendentalist Amos Bronson Alcott, who, in turn, was the father of Louisa May. During the early nineteenth century, Graham and Alcott began to preach the virtues of unadulterated brown bread and vegetarianism, the promotion of health and self-reliance, the avoidance of chemical medicine and medical doctors and the maintenance of a virtuous lifestyle. They were what Whorton calls 'physiological missionaries' who promised 'the kingdom of health' (Whorton, 1982). While the two men were generally in accord, this is not to say that there were no disagreements between them. For example, William Alcott opposed the use of yeast, the mixing of cereals and the use of salad greens (Fuller, 1989, p. 292); his cousin Amos Bronson Alcott forbade his followers all dark 'base' vegetables that grew under the ground (Roe, 1986); Graham, on the other hand, was relatively moderate and concentrated instead on promoting abstinence from alcohol and sex. Despite these family and friendly squabbles, they all advocated 'natural' vegetarian diets and healthy living as the foundation and precondition for Christian living. Coarse whole-grain bread was their symbol of purity and righteousness. Collectively they represented a movement of 'Christian physiologists express[ing] a terrestrial Edenic theme within their religion of nature' (Albanese, 1990).

In 1863, at his health reform sanatorium in upstate New York, James Caleb Jackson (originally a militant Christian abolitionist), concocted what he called 'granula' from Graham flour (Cayleff, 1987; Money, 1985; Nissenbaum, 1980; Schwartz, 1980). Eating this 'pure' food, he argued would not only prepare a person for the Second Coming but also hasten its arrival. This early granola promoted calmness, Christian morality and a disposition for progressive politics, even, as it reduced carnal desire. It was imbued with a Graham–Alcott sense of nature which, in addition to being Christian (of the anti-Calvinist persuasion) and against medical doctors, was also 'against the enslavement of the African race, against the domestic enslavement of women and against the economic enslavement of laborer' (Whorton, 1975, p. 475).

John Harvey Kellogg (1852–1943), of cornflakes fame, himself a Seventh Day Adventist, reintroduced granola in 1878 at his Battle Creek Sanatorium (Kellogg changed the spelling because of a legal suit (Nissenbaum, 1980)). Now the grahamite cereal became a dietary symbol of the temperate vision and distinct conservative style of the founding prophetess of Seventh Day Adventism, Ellen G. White (Numbers, 1972). 'Natural' living for the Adventist was like the Saturday sabbath, it helped to set a person apart from the mainstream Christian world. At the same time, it served to refine the individual and create a community in preparation for the Second Coming. Later, Kellogg, who was the leading health food advocate and natural healer of the late nineteenth century moved towards a Mind Cure position, which believed 'positive thought' promoted 'good health'. From this new perspective as an ex-Adventist, Kellogg argued that granola cultivated a harmonious interpenetration of mind and body (Deutsch, 1977; Whorton, 1988).

The next chapter in the history of granola was authored by Bernarr MacFadden (1868–1955). MacFadden was the leading, and most commercial, 'drugless therapist' of the early twentieth century and his ideas continued to exercise an influence over the movement until past the middle of the century through such students as Charles Atlas (aka Angelo Siciliano), Paul Bragg, Jack Lalane and J.I. Rodale (aka J.I. Cohen) (Whorton, 1989). Whereas earlier versions of granola had been intended to facilitate abstinence and Christian morality, MacFadden's Nature and his granola (which he called 'strength-fude', again to avoid a legal suit) exemplified a distinctly new message. Exactly 67 years after James Caleb Jackson's culinary invention of granula at his health reform sanatorium in upstate New York, MacFadden – who now owned that very resort – played host to 40 cadets sent by Mussolini from the Fascist University in Rome to study a 'natural' approach to virility, brute physical power and other he-man virtues (Ernst, 1991). In other words, MacFadden's 'natural' granola had come to be associated with the cultivation of a secular, aggressive, muscular Nature, which even had eugenic and racist overtones (Schwartz, 1970). Instead of prescribing granola to diminish lustful desire, MacFadden promoted it as a food that would develop a powerful, brute nature. To supplement its effects, he added the use of 'peniscopes' to enlarge the male organ, and breast development devices (Harrison, 1987, p. 299).

It is of interest that macrobiotics had a similar right-wing outlook during this time. In 1939, George Ohsawa, the main creative formulator of macrobiotics, toured Manchuria, supported the 'Great East Asian Co-Prosperity Sphere' and called for academic purges in medicine and science for those who did not support 'Blud und Boden' (blood and soil) medicine. Later, Ohsawa made a complete reversal, advocated peace and was imprisoned and tortured by the Japanese government. By 1949, Ohsawa had significantly reduced the specifically Japanese national component of the diet and was open to other perspectives including socialism (Frances, 1976; Kotzsch, 1981).

As usual, the possible meaning of natural food was flexible enough to allow widely disparate appropriation during the early twentieth century. Groups as different as left-wing socialists like the early Fabians (Twigg, 1979) and right-wingers like MacFadden and even some of the Nazi leadership (Barkas, 1975; Unshuld, 1980) could adopt the symbols of Nature or vegetarianism as proof and practice of their movements of social regeneration.

By the time granola and vegetarianism were reintroduced in the 'holistic' wave of the 1960s, they had become enmeshed in a now more psychological America and were associated with the human potential movement, self-fulfilment and self-awareness (Wallis, 1985). Granola's natural vision now supported various sexual options and preferences, and was associated with promoting sensitivity and deep feelings. Natural food had, again, become more clearly politically progressive. The 1965 rescinding of the Asian Exclusion Act increased Asian immigration to the United States and coincided with increased American attraction to the East. Influenced by Asia (Kandel and Pelto, 1980), the new vegetarians of the 1960s (Dwyer *et al.*, 1973), introduced yin and yang (Kotzsch, 1981) and the Indian Ayurvedic Tri-Doshas into the wholesome grain dialogue (Lad, 1984; Svoboda, 1988). East Asian and Hindu dietary regimes along with their accompanying religious ideas, became forces in dietary reform (Kandel and Pelto, 1980). Christian and secular muscles were relegated to the margins of the dietary reform movement. The post-1960s holistic movement updated the long-standing American dietary reform tradition of Nature, vegetarianism and social regeneration with psychology, renewed progressive politics and Eastern ideas and spirituality.

SYMBOL, MEDICINE AND MORALITY

The symbolic code and ethical implications of Nature and health food, although changing through history, is somehow always evident to participants (Cody, 1985). Moral beliefs somehow are always reflected in the unprocessed grains and beans. Adherence to special diets and lifestyles allows for a distinct embodiment of virtue. Values and morality, in other words, are given physical form.* Health is a moral status, getting well 'transform[s] individual hygiene

---

*Scholars have noted that moral values are encoded in any medical system. 'When we analyse physicians' concepts of, say, disease, we find in spite of the scientific gloss, that their moral value, social attitudes or political prejudices are deeply embedded in their knowledge' (Gabby, 1982). J. Comaroff makes a similar point: 'medical knowledge presents as "natural" what is actually a culturally constituted and socially motivated image of man' (1982).

into a moral–social crusade' (Whorton, 1982). Instead of the ambiguity and uncertainty of disease, health reform provides a clear and cogent path. A person's body and health are transformed into the arena of the cosmic restoration of a 'kingdom of health'. A new daily routine connects a person to a natural world that is different from the 'artificial' world of human-created culture. Regular society is contaminated and corrupt; it has disease; Nature is the source of purity, authenticity and health. Disease is immorality; nature is morality. When sickness threatens a person's survival and viability, alternative health reform reconnects him or her to a world without blemishes, imperfection or disease. Health reform is salvation by physiology, a therapeutic morality ritual. 'The dietary laws' are what Mary Douglas, speaking in another context, calls 'signs which at every turn inspired meditation on . . . oneness [and] purity . . . Observance of the dietary rules would thus have been a meaningful part of [a] great liturgical act of recognition' (Douglas, 1966). Radical health reform, for many people, is a compelling alternative offering a persuasive rationale and comprehensive practice in the face of the disruption, disorder and uncertainty of sickness.

CURRENT STATUS

The dividing line between alternative dietary reform and conventional nutrition used to be clearer than it is now. Nineteenth-century medicine, lacking knowledge of such health factors as vitamins and fibre, was inclined to see meat and potatoes as the best food, sometimes even holding vegetables and fruit in contempt (Ackerknect, 1973). The leading scientific nutritional authority of the last part of the nineteenth century suggested that wheat bran and potato skins were 'refuse' (Harrison, 1987, p. 142) However, the recent advocacy of low fat, high fibre, cruciferous vegetables and so on, within conventional medicine has blurred the demarcation. Regular restaurants offer vegetarian entrées, and granola itself has penetrated the conventional supermarket. The discovery of the role of such substances as asgenistein, indoles, limonoids, linolenic acid and lycopene all derived from vegetables and fruits, is likely to erode further the distinction between alternative and conventional dietary approaches. In retrospect, it could be said that Graham and Kellogg and their modern representatives advocated some ideas ahead of their time (McGuire, 1988). Nonetheless, certain differences between conventional nutrition and alternative dietary regimes persist. The most important of these is that unconventional dietary reform will continue to carry its overtones of a moral crusade. Alternative dietary lifestyles will probably continue the 'search for perfect bodily purity and/or moral consistency' using a 'populist physiological polemic'. (Harrison, 1987) that wraps alternative medical therapy in a persuasive moralist package.

ACKNOWLEDGEMENTS

The author wishes to thank the John E. Fetzer Institute for its support and Linda Barnes for her suggestions.

REFERENCES

Ackerknect, H.E. (1973) A history of diet, in *Therapeutics: From the Primitives to the Twentieth Century*, Hafner, New York, pp. 179–87.

Albanese, C.L. (1990) *Nature Religion in America*, University of Chicago Press, Chicago, IL.

Anderson, M.A. (1975) Nutritional knowledge of health food users in Oahu, Hawaii. *Journal of the American Dietetic Association*, **67**, 118.

Anon. (1989) Unproven methods of cancer management: macrobiotic diets for the treatment of cancer. *CA–A Cancer Journal for Clinicians*, **39**(4), 248–250.

Barkas, J. (1975) *The Vegetable Passion: A History of the Vegetarian State of Mind*, Routledge & Kegan Paul, London.

Beckford, J.A. (1984) Holistic imagery and ethics in new religious and healing movements. *Social Compass*, **31**(2–3), 265.

Bircher-Benner, M. (1959) *Prevention from Incurable Disease*, Clarke, Cambridge.

Bloomfield, R.J. (1983) Naturopathy, in *Traditional Medicine and Health Care Coverage* (eds Bannerman *et al.*), World Health Organization, Geneva, p. 121.

Bowman, B.B. *et al.* (1984) Macrobiotic diets for cancer treatment and prevention. *Journal of Clinical Oncology*, **2**, 702–11.

Brown, J.H. *et al.* (1980) Unorthodox treatments in rheumatoid arthritis. *Arthritis and Rheumatism*, **23**, S657.

Cassileth, B.R. *et al.* (1984) Contemporary unorthodox treatments in cancer medicine. *Annals of Internal Medicine*, **101**, 105–12.

Caylett, S.E. (1987) *Wash and Be Healed: The Water-Cure Movement and Women's Health*, Temple University Press, Philadelphia, PA, pp. 94, 115.

Cody, G. (1985) History of naturopathic medicine, in *A Textbook of Natural Medicine*, (eds J.F. Pizzornoa and M.J. Murray), John Bastyr College Publications, Seattle, WA, p. 10.

Comaroff, J. (1982) Medicine; symbol and ideology, in *The Problem of Medical Knowledge* (eds P. Wright and A. Treacher), Edinburgh University Press, Edinburgh, p. 52.

Coward, R. (1989) *The Whole Truth: The Myth of Alternative Health*, Faber & Faber, London.

Cowart, V.S. (1988) Health fraud's toll: lost hopes, misspent billions. *Journal of the American Dietetic Association*, **259**(22), 3229–30.

Cronan, T.A., *et al.* (1989) Prevalence of the use of unconventional remedies for arthritis in a metropolitan community. *Arthritis and Rheumatism*, **32**, 12.

Deutsch, R.M. (1970) *The New Nuts Among the Berries*, Deutsch, Palo Alto, CA, p. 80.

Douglas, M. (1966) *Purity and Danger*, Routledge & Kegan Paul, London.

Dubisch, J. (1981) You are what you eat: religious aspects of the health food movement, in *The American Dimension: Cultural Myths and Social Realities*, Alfred Publishing, Sherman Oaks, CA, p. 122.

Dwyer, J.T. (1973) The new vegetarians. *Journal of the American Dietetic Association*, **62**, 503–9.

Dyer, J.C. (1982) *Vegetarianism: An Annotated Bibliography*, Scarecrow Press, Metuchen, NJ.

Ehret, A. (1953) *Mucusless-Diet Healing System*. Ehret Literature, Cody, NY.

Eisenberg, D.M. *et al.* (1993) Unconventional medicine in the United States. *New England Journal of Medicine*, **328**, 246–52.

Ernst, R. (1991) *Weakness is a Crime: The Life of Bernard MacFadden*, Syracuse University Press, Syracuse, NY, p. 103.

Frances, K.R. (1976) Rice, ice cream and the guru: decision-making and innovation in a macrobiotic community. PhD dissertation, City University of New York, New York.

Fried, J. (1984) *Vitamin Politics*, Prometheus Books, Buffalo, NY.

Fuller, R.C. (1989) *Alternative Medicine and American Religious Life*, Oxford University Press, New York.

Gabby, J. (1982) Asthma attacked? Tactics for the reconstruction of a disease concept, in *The Problem of Medical Knowledge* (eds P. Wright and A. Treacher), Edinburgh University Press, Edinburgh, p. 23.

Gevitz, N. (1988) Three perspectives on unorthodox medicine, in *Other Healers: Unorthodox Medicine in America* (ed. N. Gevitz), John Hopkins University Press, Baltimore, MD, pp. 1–28.

Gifft, H.H. and Washbon, M.B. (1972) Nutrition, behavior and change. Prentice Hall, Englewood Cliffs, NJ, p. 91.

Green, H. (1986) *Fit for America: Health, Fitness, Sports and American Society*, The Johns Hopkins University Press, Baltimore, MD, p. 10–13.

Gutman, H.G. (1973) Work, culture and society in industrializing American, 1815–1919. *American History Review*, **78**, 531–88.

Harris & Associates (1987) Health, information and the use of questionable treatments: a study of the American public. Department of Health and Human Services, Washington, DC.

Harrison, J.F.C. (1987) Early Victorian radicals and the medicine fringe, in *Medical Fringe and Medical Orthodoxy 1750–1850* (eds W.F. Bynum and R. Porter), Croom Helm, London, pp. 216–33.

Herbert, V. (1980) The vitamin craze. *Annals of Internal Medicine*, **140**, 173–6.

Herbert, V. and Barrett, S. (1981) *Vitamins and 'Health' Foods: The Great American Hustle*, George F. Stickley, Philadelphia, PA, p. 99.

Hoff, H.E. and Fulton, J.F. (1973) The centenary of the first American physiological society founded at Boston by William A. Alcott and Sylvester Grahan. *Bulletin of the History of Medicine*, **5**(8), 703, 710.

Hongladeron, G.C. (1976) Health seeking within the health food movement. PhD dissertation, University of Washington, p. 5.

Jukes, T.H. (1977) Organic food. *CRC Critical Reviews in Food Science and Nutrition*, (November).

Kandel, R.F. and Pelto, G.H. (1980) The health food movement: social revitalization or alternative health maintenance system? in *Nutritional Anthropology: Contemporary Approaches to Diet and Culture* (eds N.W. Jerome *et al.*), Redgrave, Pleasantville, NY.

Kotzsch, R.E. (1981) George Ohsawa and the Japanese religious traditions: a study of the life and thought of the founder of macrobiotics. PhD dissertation, Harvard University Press, Cambridge, MA.

Kronenfeld, J.J. and Wasner, C. (1982) The use of unorthodox therapies and marginal practitioners. *Social Science in Medicine*, **16**, 1122.

Kulvinskas, V. (ed) (1981) *Life in the Twenty-First Century*, Omangod Press, Woodstock Valley, CT.

Lad, V. (1984) *Ayurveda: The Science of Self-Healing*, Lotus, Santa Fe, NM, p. 99A–99B.

Lane, I.W. and Comac, L. (1992) *Sharks Don't Get Cancer*, Avery, Garden City Park, NY.

McGuire, M.B. (1988) *Ritual Healing in Suburban America*, Rutgers University Press, New Brunswick, NJ, p. 99.

Mogadam, M. (1990) Nutritional fads. *American Journal of Gastroenterology*, **85**(3), 510–15.

Money, F. (1985) *The Destroying Angel: Sex, Fitness and Food in the Legacy of Degeneracy Theory, Graham Crackers, Kellogg's Corn Flakes and American Health History*, Prometheus Books, Buffalo, NY, p. 21.

New, P.K.M. and Priest, R.P. (1967) Food and thought: a sociologic study of food cultists. *Journal of the American Dietetic Association*, **51**, 13–18.

Nissenbaum, S. (1980) *Sex, Diet and Debility in Jacksonian America: Sylvester Graham and Health Reform*, Greenwood Press, Westport, CT, p. 170.

Numbers, R.L. (1992) *Prophetess for Health: Ellen G. White and the Origins of Seventh-Day Adventist Health Reform*, University of Tennessee Press, Knoxville, TN.

Read, M.H. *et al.* (1989) Health beliefs and supplement use: adults in seven western states. *Journal of the American Dietetic Association*, **89**, 1812–13.

Roe, D.A. (1986) History of promotion of vegetable cereal diets. *Journal of Nutrition*, **116**, 1355–63.

Schwartz, R. (1970) *John Harvey Kellogg, M.D.*, Southern Publishing, Nashville, TN, p. 24.

Svoboda, R.E. (1988) Prakruti: *Your Ayurvedic Constitution*. Geocom, Albuquerque, NM, pp. 64–70.

Taylor, T. (1965) Introduction, in *Porphry: On Abstinence from Animal Food*. (ed. E. Wynne-Tyson), Centaur Press, p. 15.

Todhunter, E.N. (1973) Food habits, food faddism and nutrition. *Food, Nutrition and Health. World Review of Nutrition and Dietetics*, **16**, 286–317.

Twigg, J. (1979) Food for thought: purity and vegetarianism. *Religion*, **9**, 13–33.

US Congress, Office of Technology Assessment (1990) *Unconventional Cancer Treatments*, OTA-H-405, US Government Printing Office, Washington, DC, p. 59–66.

Unshuld, P.U. (1980) The issue of structured coexistence of scientific and alternative medical systems: a comparison of East and West German legislation. *Social Science in Medicine*, **14B**, 17.

Wallis, R. (1985) Betwixt therapy and salvation: the changing form of the human potential movement, in *Sickness and Sectarianism* (ed. R.K. Jones), Gower, Aldershot.

Warner, J.H. (1978) 'The Nature-trusting heresy': American physicians and the concept of the healing power of nature in the 1850's and 1860's. *Perspectives in American History*, **11**, 291.

White, H.S. (1972) The organic foods movement. *Food Technology*, (April), 29–33.

Whorton, J. C. (1975) 'Christian physiology': William Alcotts's prescription for the millennium. *Bulletin of the History of Medicine*, **49**, 466–81.

Whorton, J.C. (1982) *Crusaders for Fitness: The History of American Health Reformers*, Princeton University Press, Princeton, NJ.

Whorton, J.C. (1988) Patient, heal thyself: popular health reform movements as unorthodox medicine, in *Other Healers: Unorthodox Medicine in America* (ed. N. Gevitz), Johns Hopkins University Press, Baltimore, MD.

Whorton, J.C. (1989) The first holistic revolution: alternative medicine in the nineteenth century, in *Examining Holistic Medicine* (eds D. Stalker and C. Glymour), Prometheus Books, Buffalo, NY.

The myth of Bach

2

Saul Berkovitz

INTRODUCTION

One of the distinguishing features of complementary medicine is the development of healing systems, either by radical and charismatic pioneers in apparent isolation, or as a reflection of broader social movements. The prevalence of these healing systems may be due to the tenacity of a small group of loyal followers or to a 'rediscovery' at a later date, sometimes by nostalgic individuals or groups in periods of perceived social crisis. This process may result in the system persisting in a fossilised form, with excessive reverence for its founder's every tenet, no matter how idiosyncratic or constrained by cultural or historical factors. A conflict may develop between 'progressive' and 'reactive' adherents, or the field may fragment into warring factions divided by subtle differences in interpretation of earlier authorities, in much the same way as religious groups. As with the latter, the smaller the numbers involved, the more bitter the fighting, the lower the quality of argument and the more hindrance to positive and progressive development.

Conventional medicine involves a model of linear progress, with outmoded ideas being discarded for new ones in response to accumulating evidence. It is of particular interest that the opinions of individual authorities exert relatively little influence. Historical reference is now made only to 'pioneers' of an approach (Semmelweis, Lind), to the opening up of new fields of inquiry (Crick and Watson, Fleming), or as the examiner's dreaded question in relation to an eponymous disease ('Hmm . . . and just who *was* Parkinson?'). Even the father of medicine, Hippocrates, would be unlikely to merit a mention in today's medical school curriculum, whereas, for instance, it would be unusual to find a contribution to the homoeopathic literature making no reference to Hahnemann, Hering or Kent.

The changing of views in orthodox medicine is, in theory, restrained by questions of scientific validity and reproducibility, as well as by natural conservatism, but no longer by appeal to individual authority. The situation in some branches of complementary medicine is rather different. This chapter takes a look at the history of one such system, the 'Flower Remedies' of Edward Bach (pronounced 'batch'), in which the figure of Bach looms large, and in which myth making has played a prominent part. I examine the history given by the current authorities, compare this to an account obtained by historical scholarship and attempt to identify the function served by what I see as a mythologising of the life of Bach.

HISTORY OF BACH AND HIS REMEDIES

Bach was by most accounts a successful bacteriologist and Harley Street physician in the 1920s and 1930s. He had leanings towards homoeopathy and eventually abandoned his lucrative practice and began wandering the British countryside in search of healing herbs, eventually developing a spiritualised system of medicine based on the effects of preparations of wild flowers on various states of mind. He settled in an idyllic hamlet in Oxfordshire, where, upon his death at 50 in 1936, the legacy of his work was bequeathed to two devoted lay adherents, Nora Weeks and Victor Bullen. Their tenacity in maintaining what was literally a cottage industry and practice has paid dividends over the last decade with the upsurge of interest in complementary medicine. Bach's remedies are now manufactured on a massive scale by Nelson's, the homoeopathic pharmaceuticals company, and distributed worldwide in a multi-million pound market with competition from numerous other 'Flower Remedy' systems, notably Australian and Californian. The cottage (now the Bach Centre) in Sotwell, near Didcot, has become a teaching centre for Bach practitioners as well as a place of pilgrimage for those seeking spiritual enlightenment.

The life of Bach proves difficult to reconstruct with any accuracy. The only available biography is a slim volume written by Nora Weeks (1940), which, being written for the benefit of Flower Remedy users, concentrates on his search for the Remedies during the last ten years of his life. The account is notable for its paucity of biographical detail and consistently betrays a tendency towards hagiography. None of his colleagues is still alive (Nora Weeks and Victor Bullen both died in the 1970s), and other information is purely apocryphal. In addition, much of the material concerning Bach's transition from relative orthodoxy to the very fringe of his profession was supposedly destroyed in a large bonfire that Bach made of his work before leaving London on his quest, a pyromaniac tendency repeated several times over the next few years as his system neared 'perfection'. Only a few letters and a single photograph of a well groomed and professionally posed Bach (who 'hated having his photo taken') were salvaged. The dearth of historical source material is itself an important part in the creation of a legend. Bach's only surviving possessions, proudly displayed in the front room of the Bach Centre, are three bottles of tinctures and a few simple pieces of self-made furniture. Bach's death occasioned only one short obituary notice in a homoeopathic journal (*British Homoeopathic Journal*, 1937), and none in orthodox journals. His published work was sparse (deliberately so in latter years): a few papers in orthodox journals and later in homoeopathic journals; one small work, *Chronic Disease* (1925), summarising his bacteriological research, and two pamphlets concerned with his Flower Remedies; *Heal Thyself* (1931), his spiritualist philosophy of life; and *The Twelve Healers and Other Remedies* (1933), the final version of his pharmacopoeia containing 38 remedies and their indications. Previous versions are kept in the Centre's archives but not released 'at his own request' so as not to disrupt the 'purity and simplicity' of the complete system. This, as we shall see, distracts attention from the evolution of Bach's ideas, which might have been ongoing, and creates an image of a static, fully formed system with no possibility of further development.

Nora Weeks' role in creating the myth of Bach is clear from the language of her short biography, *The Medical Discoveries of Edward Bach, Physician* (1940). Weeks was a radiographer, who met Bach in 1929 and became his 'closest helper, companion and chosen successor'. She presents an image of Bach as a visionary genius, a wise teacher possessed of an 'inner knowledge'. The historiography is heavily laden with overtones of predetermination, insisting that Bach's destiny from birth was his search for a 'simple certain cure for disease', fulfilled at last by his discovery of the Flower Remedies. Details of Bach's personal, social and professional life are sketchy; there is no mention at all of his mother, names of parents or siblings, his two marriages, his medical colleagues or, most surprisingly, even of Weeks herself. It is as if Bach's life takes place in a vacuum, focused entirely on his divinely inspired quest to cure the ills of humankind.

Three themes are stressed in regard to Bach's early life: his personal qualities of 'genius' and 'intensity of purpose', his 'overwhelming compassion' for fellow beings whether human or animal and his 'love of Nature', taking long rambles 'happy in the company of his friends the birds and trees and wild flowers'. A sense of destiny runs through his childhood: 'he knew his life's work from the start', possessing 'inner knowledge of what was to come', and was already aware of his natural healing abilities. The only other account of Bach's life available, Julian Barnard's *Patterns of Life Force* (1987), talks of the care the young Bach took of his siblings and the weak and needy. Similar features are found in other hagiographies of leading figures in complementary medicine, for example, Trevor Cook's biography of Hahnemann.

Bach is said to have left school at 16 and worked for three years in his father's brass foundry. The reason Weeks gives for this surprising turn of events reflects further glory on Bach: 'he felt he could not ask them (his parents) to stand the expense of his long training'; Barnard suggests 'false modesty', 'pride, fear, lack of confidence', 'indecision', and conflict with parental expectations. Bach eventually entered Birmingham University in 1906 at the age of 20, and University College Hospital (UCH), London, in 1909. His tireless study is said to have been hampered only by his yearning for the countryside, which forced him to avoid the London parks in case 'the call of Nature proved too strong'. Bach is portrayed on a threadbare allowance, taking odd jobs, correcting exam papers and even going hungry to buy textbooks. This is inconsistent, since according to Weeks, Bach had little use for books, preferring to spend hours at the bedside observing individual cases.

He qualified in 1912, then took the Diploma of Public Health in 1914. Having been refused for war service on account of fragile health, Bach became Assistant Bacteriologist at UCH under Francis Teale (1875–1959), a distinguished bacteriologist known for his work on meningococcal meningitis. Bach's career direction at this time certainly does not accord with his intuitive healing gift and his mission to find 'a simple, certain cure for disease'. Three papers bearing the names of Teale and Bach appear in the *Proceedings of the Royal Society of Medicine* (1919–1920), the only time the latter's work reached an orthodox journal. They are concerned with techniques in bacterial cultures, and are of little importance. They are not, as Weeks asserts, connected with his work on therapeutic vaccines, which never achieved publication in a medical journal. This error is significant because Bach's vaccine work is continually adduced to emphasise his standing in the scientific community of the time.

Indeed, the notable feature of Bach's life during this period is not his medical achievements but his health; in July 1917 he 'had a severe haemorrhage and became unconscious', requiring emergency surgery. The nature of this illness is uncertain, though Weeks intimates (and Barnard asserts) that it was cancer. Bach's death certificate 19 years later cited 'primary cardiac failure and sarcoma', possibly a recurrence of this earlier illness. Weeks ascribes the disease to Bach 'working unceasingly, giving himself no rest, and fainting at the laboratory bench'. Clearly Bach's personal life was in turmoil at the time: his wife of four years died of diphtheria in April 1917, yet one month later he remarried and registered the birth of the new couple's 15-month-old daughter. They were to separate a few years later. Bach's later shortcomings as a father are notable in view of his strongly and persistently expressed liberal views on the raising of children.

Bach's recovery is described in suitably heroic language: desperate to fulfil his destiny in the remaining three months prognosticated by his surgeon, Bach struggled up from his death bed back to his work bench. Immersing himself in research, 'he forgot his own disabilities and found himself growing stronger', astounding his colleagues. However, during the following year he left UCH in a dispute over private practice. Weeks' explanation is Bach's 'dislike for rules and regulations', though financial considerations must have played a part since the salaries offered by the medical school were minimal and most of the staff undertook private work to supplement their wages.

BACH'S WORK ON BACTERIAL VACCINES – 'NOSODES'

By 1920 Bach could boast a consulting room in Harley Street and a private bacteriology laboratory. He had also been appointed as pathologist at the Royal London Homoeopathic Hospital, possibly due to the influence of Teale, who was a friend of Sir John Weir, physician to royalty and a leading figure in the British Homoeopathic Society. This association resulted in Teale's regularly attending and delivering lectures at Society meetings. It was here that Bach read Hahnemann's *Organon*, the bible of homoeopathy, which promised individualised, safe treatment (Hahnemann, 1982). He emphasised the similarities between this and his own methods in a paper presented to the Society, entitled 'The relation of vaccine therapy to homoeopathy' (Bach, 1920). Bach apparently faced resistance among homoeopaths over the incorporation of his relatively orthodox methods as he tried to build up the 'long neglected' Bacteriology Department. This perhaps accounts for his obsequious introduction to the paper: 'May I present my allopathic offering at the altar of your science'. However, Bach did extend the work of his department and continued to experiment with his vaccines, now prepared homoeopathically and known as the Bach nosodes.

In 1922 the pressure of routine work at the hospital began to interfere with his research and he left, going back to Harley Street and his new laboratory in Park Crescent, Portland Place, a row of buildings occupied entirely by private practitioners using many unorthodox therapies. His vaccine work was published as 'Chronic disease: a working hypothesis' in 1926 in collaboration with Charles Wheeler, a physician at the Royal London Homoeopathic Hospital. Bach's interest in vaccine therapy dates from about ten years earlier, during his time at University College, where he prepared vaccines based on certain intestinal bacteria isolated from patients, normally considered non-pathogenic but which he felt to be associated with chronic diseases. Unfortunately, the technique of vaccine therapy promulgated by physicians such as Sir Almroth Wright, and the doctrine of faecal autointoxication, promoted by the no less colourful William Arbuthnot Lane (both men merited mention in Bernard Shaw's farce *The Doctor's Dilemma*), had both been under fire during Bach's ten years of labour (Foster, 1970; *Lancet*, 1922). The time was over-ripe for Bach's work, and reaction was muted. A cursory review in the *British Medical Journal* adopted a sceptical tone, lamenting the lack of 'convincing evidence to warrant the bad character' given to the offending bacteria, and disdaining the excellent clinical results quoted. There is no evidence to back up Bach's claim that 'hundreds of homoeopaths and allopaths were achieving marvellous results' with the vaccines, or Weeks' statement that 'they were enthusiastically welcomed by the medical profession'.

Among homoeopaths, however, initial reaction was favourable. The British Homoeopathic Society was anxious to claim Bach's work for itself (*British Homoeopathic Journal*, 1925). This was in spite of the fact that the book discreetly avoided any direct mention of homoeopathy, and the method of administration suggested was that of injection rather than the oral, homoeopathic version that Bach had developed five years earlier. (Bach was acutely conscious that a potentised 'nosode' would be too 'homoeopathic' for orthodox physicians to swallow (Bach, 1927). Bach hovered uneasily between orthodoxy and homoeopathy: from 1922 he was without an official post, remaining a Harley Street physician with a private laboratory. He was aware that to identify publicly with homoeopathy would alienate the profession, and prevent his work reaching the larger medical world. By 1929 he had come to believe that his work would be more safely guarded and likely to survive among homoeopaths. Ironically, the initial enthusiasm was already waning. Distinguished homoeopaths such as Sir John Weir and Douglas Borland found the nosodes 'not much use' or 'merely a tonic' (Gordon, 1936), and Bach was forced into an extraordinary outburst in which he pleaded for his work to be 'watched and directed by the homoeopathic school, and not be allowed to fall into the hands of men [the allopaths] who do not understand the fundamental principles on which it is based' (Bach, 1929). It was left to John Paterson, a Scottish homoeopath, to translate Bach's work into something more palatable to homoeopaths, such as a list of appropriate indications to prescribe a standard remedy – instead of isolating bacteria from the patient's faeces (Paterson, 1950).

BACH'S CHANGING PHILOSOPHY AND THE DEVELOPMENT OF THE FLOWER REMEDIES

By the late 1920s Bach's reputation was at its peak. But he remained dissatisfied, both by the limited scope of use of his therapeutic vaccines or nosodes, and by his wish to replace them with 'purer' herbal remedies. This wish appears to have been driven not by his own desire, as Weeks suggests, but by the reluctance of homoeopaths to use his bacterial nosodes. Irritated at having to satisfy 'the aesthetic mentality of the most fastidious type', he began experimenting with herbs from 1928, and formulated a philosophy of health and disease which concentrated increasingly on mental and emotional factors. Although Weeks is adamant that this was Bach's 'destiny' from birth, it should be noted that she only met him in 1929, after he had developed similar views on predestination. The available evidence suggests that his change of direction occurred between 1928 and 1930. He had become interested in healing methods such as electricity, X-rays and the 'Adams Box' (a radionic device supposed to emit healing rays of unknown type), and had worked with the clairvoyant Geoffrey Hodgson (Richards, 1934), to whose book *A New Light on Health and Disease* (1929) his own pamphlet *Heal Thyself* (1930) bears a remarkable resemblance. However, Weeks' assertion that as early as 1922 Bach was 'working out the "mentals" or personality types in each of whom one of the seven bacterial groups predominated', is far-fetched; he consistently advocated stool cultures rather than symptomatology until the late 1920s. Even in 1930, his first and only list of clinical indications for prescribing his nosodes is a terse affair (produced in response to the homoeopaths' demands), and does not lay undue stress on mental symptoms (Bach, 1930).

His new outlook first appears in print in a lecture given to the Southport Homoeopathic Debating Society in October 1929 (Bach, 1930), Southport being the home of Dr F.J. Wheeler, one of the few homoeopaths to follow Bach's new vision. The lecture reveals a messianic fervour quite unlike any of his previous writings: he railed against the decadence of modern medicine (in particular the practice of Voronoff whose anti-ageing therapy involved transplanting monkey testicle to the human scrotum); paraded the wisdom of the ancients of India and China, kept alive only by Hippocrates, Paracelsus, Culpeper and Hahnemann; and maintained that disease stems from spiritual error alone. He also hinted that 'several new remedies have been discovered, some of which are found to be working on the mental plane rather than the physical . . . these will make homoeopathy such a power in the world that nothing will withstand it'. This intense and poetic use of language marks all his later writings, and must have been a great inspiration to his followers. The indications for the remedies described, however, show a mixture of homoeopathic, allopathic and mental features, indicating that Bach's ideas were still evolving. Interestingly, two of the five remedies were not prepared from wild flowers. These were omitted in Weeks' account.

In 1930 Bach left London to search for herbal remedies in the countryside. The results were published, not in the rather conservative *British Homoeopathic Journal* (which distanced itself from his philosophy) but in *Homoeopathic World*, the populist magazine of the British Homoeopathic Association, between December 1930 and June 1931. Pamphlets were also published through C.W. Daniel, a small publishing outlet specialising in alternative health and esoteric philosophy. These articles enlarged upon Bach's philosophy, extended his list of remedies and introduced the 'sun' method of preparation, which involved placing flower blooms in a glass bowl full of water in a sunny field and allowing the sun to transmit their healing energy into the water. To 'preserve' the elixir, he would half-fill several small bottles, making them up with household brandy. The resulting 'tincture' would be prescribed as a couple of drops to a glass of water. (The crateloads of brandy delivered to the cottage in Sotwell became a standing joke among the villagers, especially in view of Bach's well known partiality to alcohol.) Weeks describes the discovery of this method as a stroke of inspiration about the potency of the dew on the flowers. However, he would have known of Paracelsus 'gathering the dew under varying configurations of the heavenly bodies, believing the water to carry with it the energy of the planetary influences' (Tompkins and Bird, 1973). In addition, he had already made mention of astrology as a useful consideration in the gathering of herbs (Bach, 1930).

Later editions of the remedies show a graded change to 'mentally' based prescribing. For instance, in *The Twelve Healers and Seven Helpers* (Bach, 1934) remedies were reclassified according to the patient's physical complexion. Bach used several different methods to decide on appropriate flowers for various states of mind (usually determined in advance): aesthetic beauty, the doctrine of signatures, mediumship, folklore and even enquiring about patients' own preferences. Bach's followers claim that he began to develop disturbing physical symptoms as his senses quickened, including skin rashes, leg ulcers, alopecia, temporary blindness and 'haemorrhaging', and was compelled to wander until he found the correct remedy. The intensity of this physical onslaught broke Bach's health. Inured to illness for much of his life, he felt his suffering to have been worthwhile, for the new remedies were 'even more spiritualised' than the first 19.

The reaction to Bach's spiritual theories and remedies in the homoeopathic community was one of disdain – the opposite of what Weeks would have us believe. The *British Homoeopathic Journal* noted, that 'Dr Bach seems to have stepped out of the realm of pathology and therapeutics into that of metaphysical speculation and dogmatism'(*British Homoeopathic Journal*, 1932). Esoteric societies such as the Theosophical Society welcomed his philosophical position, but ridiculed the remedies (*Theosophist*, 1931); the *Medical Herbalist* wondered whether 'the potency of the medicine is due to the herb used in preparing the tincture, or the Brandy used as a preservative?' (*Medical Herbalist*, 1933). Upon Bach's death a few years later, Charles Wheeler, his collaborator in the work on bacterial vaccines, paid tribute to his integrity, while expressing disappointment over what he saw as a wasted talent. John Paterson, who had taken over the mantle of the Bach nosodes, added a more political note by insisting that Bach 'had homoeopathy right down at the bottom of his heart' (Paterson, 1950). Bach's death passed unnoticed by the orthodox journals; in fact, his only contact with mainstream medicine in eight years had been a warning letter from the General Medical Council threatening to strike him from the Medical Register for advertising his medicines in a local newspaper (Bach then desisted and heard no more from them).

AFTER BACH: THE BACH CENTRE

The handful of Bach's followers, led by his appointed successors Nora Weeks and Victor Bullen (a builder who, impressed by Bach's healing of a friend, joined him), set about continuing 'the Work', as Bach had called it, inspired by a sense of divine purpose. They felt, and still do feel, 'provided for', 'led by an unknown hand', and cite numerous occasions on which money, flowers or other necessities have materialised when required, as if by fate. The survival and recent success of the remedies is for them a confirmation of Bach's prophecy: the 'Medicine of the Future' is now the medicine of today. From the late 1930s, interrupted only by the Second World War, Weeks saw patients in a London consulting room, and remedies were made according to Bach's method, packaged by hand at Sotwell and sent to 'friends' in England and abroad. Bach's system spread by word of mouth and through dissemination of his writings and Weeks' biography. A *Bach Remedy Newsletter* was circulated from 1952, conveying an image of cosy domesticity. A pamphlet entitled *The Story of Mount Vernon* (as the cottage at Sotwell was known) carries a full-page picture of Weeks' cat Wumps, plus anecdotes about Dr Bach's carpentry skills and Victor Bullen's glorious baritone voice (Howard, 1986). Weeks and Bullen both died in the 1970s, appointing successors after careful vetting and trial periods for their ability to uphold Bach's principles: the inheritance is kept very much 'in the family'.

The major concerns of the Bach Centre are expressed at the head of each newsletter, in a quote from Bach himself:

> Attempted distortion is a far greater weapon than attempted destruction ... As soon as a teacher has given his work to the world, a contorted version of the same must arise ... for people to be able to choose between the gold and the dross.

This is used by the Centre as an appeal (or warning) to prescribe purely on 'mental' symptoms and not, for example, by dowsing with a pendulum or by using radionic methods (despite Bach's use of radionic machines and Weeks' membership of the Society of Radionic Practitioners). It also refers to any other deviation from the final version of Bach's system. The Centre's administrators have an uncompromising attitude. They oppose the association of Bach's name with any other Flower Essences, many of which have surfaced, and have trademarked the Bach name to enable legal action to be taken against any who make such associations.

The first such extension occurred during Bach's life and occasioned the warning quoted above: a certain Dr Max Wolf suggested combining all 38 remedies in a single bottle, thus obviating the need for diagnosis of the mental state. Bach's case notes show that he had himself combined up to six remedies at a time (his 'Rescue Remedy', for shock, contains five), but he disliked the idea, perhaps influenced by Hahnemann's hatred of polypharmacy (Bach, 1990). In 1951, Alick McInnes, a psychic, marketed 'Exultation of Flowers', a remedy made by the direct transfer of healing energy from flowers to water by meditation. Since he did not use Bach's name the Centre simply dissociated itself from his product, which rapidly disappeared (*Bach Remedy Newsletter*, 1951). In 1961, Aubrey Westlake, a retired general practitioner, wrote a book that spoke of prescribing Bach remedies by radiesthetic diagnosis on a spot of blood from the patient, and introduced a 'Radiation Remedy', a composite remedy 'which Bach did not discover in his day, as nuclear radiation was still in the future'. However, he admitted that he had 'departed from the simple use of the remedies as taught by Dr. Bach', and added a testimony to the Bach Centre (Westlake, 1961), which was enough to satisfy Weeks that their territory was not threatened (*Bach Remedy Newsletter*, 1962).

Trouble flared again in the 1970s. In 1964 Weeks and Bullen had produced a book containing precise details for preparing the remedies. The intention was 'to allow people to seek and make remedies for their own healing', but Californian groups began making remedies from local non-Bach flowers, charging fees for 'field trips' and claiming to be 'the modern counterparts of Bach' (*Bach Remedy Newsletter*, 1988, 1989). Weeks, angered at these abuses, appointed a watchdog, Leslie Kaslof, to monitor the American scene, and withdrew her book from publication. In 1979 an American distributor was set up to protect the interests of the Bach Centre, and subsequently the name 'Bach Flower Remedies' was trademarked. However the strangely-named Gurudas, a Californian mystic, proved a thorn in the side of the Bach Centre. In 1983 he published *Flower Essences and Vibrational Healing* (1983), containing 112 new remedies from around the world. To justify his credentials, he claimed that Bach died without a successor, that he felt more remedies would be needed, and that his Rescue Remedy represented 'the first of many combination remedies . . . for specific imbalances'. He also cited one of Bach's own remedies, Cerato, a native Tibetan species which Bach had found growing in an English garden, to argue that the flower had to be neither native nor wild as the Bach Centre had decreed. Gurudas' esoteric philosophy (his book is 'trance-channeled' through a medium who is apparently communicating with John the Baptist) did not endear him to the Bach Centre, nor his use of dowsing, astrology and Eastern concepts such as chakras and Chinese meridians. The Centre regards him as a dangerous crank, though he is taken seriously in America.

His former colleagues Patricia Kaminski and Richard Katz have adopted a more comprehensible Steinerian 'Spiritual Science'. They argue that 'just as scientific culture can be one-sided, so can the reaction against science, whether it is in Dr. Bach's admonition, or in the New Age spiritual movement of today', and portray Bach as an empiricist with a 'systematic and disciplined approach to his work which took much from the scientific method'. Their 'professional kit' consists of 72 remedies, whose indications are expressed in similar terms to Bach's. The Bach Centre insists that his name must not be associated with them (Kaminski and Katz, 1991).

In Britain, the Bach Centre has a competitor in Julian Barnard's 'Healing Herbs', which are identical, but lack Bach's name due to trademark restrictions. Barnard is certainly a Bach purist and in 1988 was lecturing on behalf of the Bach Centre. Philosophical differences emerged, however; Barnard states that Bach's work can either be taken at face value (the Centre's attitude), or be used to 'build a bridge, taking us across to a better understanding' (Barnard, personal communication). To teach this philosophy, he set up the Bach Educational Programme, whose name had to be changed to the Flower

Remedy Programme under threat of legal action. The Bach Centre has repeatedly had to dissociate itself from Barnard and even issued a specially prepared statement to this effect.

At the centre of the arguments over proposed extensions to Bach's system have been issues such as: Did Bach appoint a rightful successor? Did he leave his system complete or allow for new remedies in a changing world? Are Bach remedies international or appropriate only for the UK? The Centre's reactions have been vigorous. Barnard is disqualified on the grounds that he has not spent time at the Centre. His remedies are stated to be lacking in potency as they have not been made at Bach's original (and secret) locations, though in practice this rule is not invariable for the Centre itself, as evidenced by the fact that they considered teaching people to make their own remedies. The Centre repeatedly insists that its administrators are the only 'lawful heirs' of Bach's work; that Bach's 38 remedies cover all possible states of mind and therefore no new remedies are needed; and that states of mind are truly universal in both time and space, which rules out any need for different remedies in different countries or in a changing world with new hazards. Here, as elsewhere, the writing about Bach implies his omnipotence, treading a thin line between fierce loyalty and outright worship as a guru figure.

> Are they really implying that Dr. Bach . . . would have been so short-sighted as to consider only the British sufferers and thereby overlook the rest of mankind? He, of all people, could not possibly be thought guilty of such an omission.
>
> *Bach Remedy Newsletter* (1988)

CONCLUSION

The mythologising of Bach seems to have served several functions. It should be noted that Bach had a tendency to mythologise himself, despite the undeniable fact that his own behaviour fell substantially short of the lofty pinnacles of his spiritualised philosophy. As we have seen, a rose-tinted view has persisted in 'official' histories of Bach, such as that by Weeks, which contrasts sharply with what we can glean of Bach's life and views from careful study of the primary sources. There are a number of reasons for the prevailing attitude:

(1) The focus on Bach's personal qualities, from his healing ability to an almost Papal infallibility, is transferred by implication to the medical system left behind: such a gifted person could not be guilty of omission or imperfection. This argument is repeatedly invoked by the Bach Centre as a defence against proposed modifications.

(2) As the Flower Remedy market has increased in value over the past two decades, commercial control has become a motivating factor, as evidenced by the copyrighting of the Bach name and the legal wrangling in

both Britain and the United States. Allied to this are issues of personal power and influence. The Bach Centre, with its internal power struggles, ruthless dismissals, expectations of blind loyalty, and hand-picked successors ('lawful heirs') has all the ingredients of a dynasty.

(3) There is a need to maintain the distinctiveness of the therapy in a rapidly expanding field. Much of the debate centres on the desire to separate use of the remedies from other vibrational therapies such as radionics, dowsing, crystal healing or homoeopathy. In one particularly interesting case in the 1970s, two members of the Bach Centre were dismissed for embracing the ideas of Rudolf Steiner, the founder of anthroposophy. This is despite the fact that both Bach and Weeks used anthroposophical medicine and that Steiner's ideas may well have influenced Bach in the 1920s.

The consequence of these attitudes is a system that has remained in stasis, fossilised in tablets of stone. Instead of critical and reflective practice, there is a blind alley. Consider the dilemma of a sensitive Bach practitioner who finds some remedies working better than others in particular situations, or when prepared from different sources or in different ways, who discovers unexpected effects of remedies, beneficial or adverse; who through clinical experience starts to question, refine or alter the existing indications (exactly as Bach did throughout his period of experimentation, which evolved continuously right up to his death). Not only is there no forum to discuss these issues, but they are dismissed as self-evidently absurd: the practitioner must be in error, even if many colleagues should encounter the same phenomena.

If, as Bach frequently averred, clinical practice is the ultimate testing ground, not textbooks or posters, then Bach Flower Remedy patients have much to gain from this type of debate. Again an analogy might be drawn with homoeopathy; although the views and works of the master, Hahnemann, in the early nineteenth century, are the starting point for education and practice, his 100 remedies have been extended to over 3000 and the original remedies refined and altered through practice. New ideas, research and philosophical formulations may be put forward in peer-reviewed journals (despite the inevitable backlash) with the result that, however chaotic the spectrum of views may seem, there is the opportunity for evolution or even major changes to the therapeutic model. The history of the Flower Remedies illustrates, in contrast, how the development of a therapeutic system can be hindered by dogmatic attitudes.

REFERENCES

Bach, E. (1920) The relation of vaccine therapy to homoeopathy. *British Homoeopathic Journal*, **10**, 67–77.

Bach, E. (1927) A note on vaccines potentised. *British Homoeopathic Journal*, **17**, 204–5.

Bach, E. (1929) The rediscovery of psora. *British Homoeopathic Journal*, **19**, 29–41.

Bach, E. (1930) Intestinal nosodes. *British Homoeopathic Journal*, **20**, 184–5.

Bach, E. (1930) Medicine of the future. *Homoeopathic World*, (February), 50–1.

Bach, E. (1930) Some fundamental considerations of disease and cure. *Homoeopathic World*, (October), 266–8.

Bach, E. (1931) *Heal Thyself*, C.W. Daniel, Saffron Walden.

Bach, E. (1933) *The Twelve Healers and Other Remedies*, C.W. Daniel, Saffron Walden.

Bach, E. (1990) Letter, in *Original Writings*, C.W. Daniel, Saffron Walden.

Bach, E. and Wheeler, C. (1925) *Chronic Disease: A Working Hypothesis*, H.K. Lewis, London.

Bach Remedy Newsletter (1951) (May); cited in Tompkins and Bird (1973) p. 275.

Bach Remedy Newsletter (1962) (March).

Bach Remedy Newsletter (1988) (August).

Bach Remedy Newsletter (1989) (August).

Barnard, J. (1987) *Patterns of Life Force*, Bach Educational Program, Hereford.

British Homoeopathic Journal (1925), **15**, 520–22.

British Homoeopathic Journal (1932) **22**, 154.

British Homoeopathic Journal (1937) **27**, 78–80.

Cook, T. *Samuel Hahnemann; His Life and Work*, Thorsons, Wellingborough.

Foster, W.D. (1970) *A History of Medical Bacteriology and Immunology*, Heinemann, London, Chapter 6, pp. 127–48.

Gordon, C. (1936) Autointoxication and psora. *British Homoeopathic Journal*, **26**, 20–30.

Gurudas (1983) *Flower Essences and Vibrational Healing*, California, p. 13.

Hahnemann, S.C. (1982) *Organon of Medicine*, 6th edn, Tarcher, Los Angeles, CA.

Hodgson, G. (1929) *A New Light on Health and Disease*, C.W. Daniel, Saffron Walden.

Howard, J. (1986) *The Story of Mount Vernon*, C.W. Daniel, Saffron Walden.

Kaminski, P. and Katz, R. (1991) *Flower Essence Society Newsletter*, (Spring).

Lancet (1922) (February).

Paterson, J. (1950) The bowel nosodes. *British Homoeopathic Journal*, **40**, 153–63.

Richards, W.G. *The Chain of Life*, p. 154.

Teale, F.H. and Bach, E. (1919–1920) The nature of serum antitrypsin and its relation to autolysis and the formation of toxins. *Proceedings of the Royal Society of Medicine*, 5–42, 43–66, 78–99, 316–32.

The Theosophist (1931) May.

Theosophist, September 1934; *Medical Herbalist* (1933) (November).

Tompkins, P. and Bird, C. (quoted in) (1973) *The Secret Life of Plants*, Allen Lane, Saffron Walden, p. 274.

Weeks, N. (1940) *The Medical Discoveries of Edward Bach, Physician*, C.W. Daniel, Saffron Walden.

Westlake, A. (1961) *The Pattern of Health*, Vincent Stuart, London.

PART TWO

Practices

This section examines the therapeutic activities of complementary practitioners. Stephen Birch argues that much of the academic debate on acupuncture involves the assumption that it is a homogeneous entity. He points out that acupuncture is extremely diverse, that no form has been shown to be superior to any other and that authors have often made simplistic assumptions about what constitutes 'correct' practice. He is particularly critical of the idea that 'traditional' acupuncture, a single coherent body of practice, unchanged for thousands of years, can be contrasted simply with 'Western' acupuncture. A similar point is made for different ends by Jeremy Swayne. Swayne argues that there are a very large number of different forms of homoeopathy. Homoeopaths vary in their overall ideology, their prescribing strategy, the dose and frequency of medications and their use of polypharmacy. There is also considerable inconsistency between different materia medica. Significant variations in practice suggest that patients are not receiving optimal care, because it is unlikely that all treatment approaches are of equivalent benefit. Peter Fisher argues that though homoeopathic prescribing is based on the use of repertories, the information they contain has never been shown to be reliable. In fact, there is good reason to doubt the provenance of many of the indications found in the repertories. Moreover, the structure of homoeopathic prescribing decisions, – i.e. the way in which homoeopaths choose one remedy over another – has not been examined sufficiently. Caroline Stevensen explores some of the beliefs and practices common among nurses interested in complementary medicine. In addition to examining key concepts such as 'holism' and 'energy', she argues that many of the therapies practised by nurses – such as massage or reflexology – have a poor research base. In particular, there is little evidence on correct indications and contra-indications or on the optimum dosages and frequencies for treatment. Bob Fordham examines the tension between the neat structure of homoeopathic 'laws' and the rather more messy world of clinical practice. He points out that therapists are often encouraged to mould perceptions of their clinical experiences so that they make sense of them in terms of homoeopathic theory. Fordham uses the example of the *dynamis*, or vital force, to illustrate this point further.

Diversity and acupuncture: acupuncture is not a coherent or historically stable tradition

3

Stephen Birch

INTRODUCTION

Since acupuncture is widely practised today and has been practised in many different social and political climates, there are naturally many ways that it has been described and practised. Many of those writing about acupuncture appear to be unaware of that diversity. In contrast to how it is described in most of the popular and professional Western literature, acupuncture is a multimodal system of healing with multiple competing explanatory models. Depending upon context, it is found as an integrated part of, a self-sufficient system of, or a discrete set of techniques within multiple systems of medical practice, both East Asian and Western origin. This essay will examine and contrast popular and more scholarly representations of acupuncture, briefly exploring reasons for some differences between them. Examples of how these differences impact on the scientific investigation of acupuncture will be presented. Finally, key issues of importance to scientists investigating acupuncture will be discussed.

BACKGROUND

Acupuncture has been practised in China for at least 2000 years, in Korea and Japan for around 1500 years, Europe for over 300 years and in North America for over 150 years (Lu and Needham, 1980). It is now practised in over 100 countries around the world (World Health Organization, 1985). It has continuously evolved since its practice began, responding to political and socio-cultural pressures, the medical exigencies of the time and the inventive creativity of individuals. This constant adaptation is partially responsible for its reception in so many periods and countries (Birch and Felt, 1997). However, it has also fostered a wide range of explanatory models, diagnostic methods, and therapeutic interventions.

Usually those involved in the study and practice of acupuncture, describe a particular explanatory model with its methods of practice. They then go on to claim (explicitly or implicitly) that what they have described is representative of the whole field. Furthermore, by suggesting that what they have described is 'correct', they imply that there is something inadequate or wrong in what others describe. We must be wary of such representations. There is therefore no historical or scientific evidence to support any claim that any particular model of acupuncture is superior to any other. Moreover, many representations about acupuncture are not entirely accurate.

In describing the history, nature and practice of acupuncture we must proceed neutrally and cautiously. I will argue that many interested in the scientific investigation of acupuncture have not been aware of these issues. They have investigated concepts or methods of questionable value and have assumed that these were representative of acupuncture as a whole. In this paper I will briefly examine the scope and nature of acupuncture, and then examine how proponents, and consequently scientists, have portrayed it. Any assessment of acupuncture should depend not only on clinical research, of which much has already been done, but also on a scholarly assessment of its nature and history. Many of the claims that have been made do not match the broader body of literature on acupuncture.

EVIDENCE FOR DIVERSITY IN ACUPUNCTURE

A comprehensive description of acupuncture is beyond the scope of this paper, but based on a review of published literature from a number of key countries we can illustrate the extent of the diversity of explanatory models and methods of practice. Table 3.1 gives examples of the varied explanatory models from China, Japan, France, the USA and the UK. While not exhaustive, it illustrates the range of models.

Proponents of particular models might take issue with the classification scheme in Table 3.1. For example, supporters of the system of 'traditional acupuncture' that is taught at the Traditional Acupuncture Institute in Columbia, Maryland, might argue that this is a traditional system and not a 'unique system'. However, no other approach attempts to meld principles and ideas from the Chinese classics with EST principles, or the American 'Human Potential Movement' of the late 1960s and early 1970s, (Cassidy, 1994); thus it is classified as unique.

Table 3.1 Examples of various explanatory models of acupuncture

	China	Japan	France	USA	UK
Traditional explanations only	Liu (1988) Wiseman (1985)	Fukushima (1991) Shudo (1990)	Larre et al. (1986)	Anon (1980) Cheng (1987)	Maciocia (1989) Worsley (1973)
Mixture of traditional and modern explanations	O'Connor and Bensky (1981)	Manaka, Itaya and Birch (1995) Nakatani and Yamashita (1977)	Mussat (1972) Requena (1986)	Helms (1995) Liao, Lee and Ng (1994)	Mann (1974)
Modern scientific explanations only		Debata (1990)		Ulett (1992)	Baldry (1989)
Unique ideas	Zhang (1979)	Suehara (1985)	Nogier (1983)	Connelly (1979) Voll (1975)	Kenyon (1983) Voll (1975)

Traditional explanatory models invoke concepts found in the earlier historical literature, many of which persist into modern practice. Examples of such concepts are the theories of: *yin-yang*, five phase, *jing-luo* (channel), *zang-fu* (organ), and *qi* (finest matter influences). Diagnostic assessments are usually stated in combinations of these terms, with treatments targeting, at least in part, those perceived problems. Modern explanations invoke concepts whose origins are typically found in modern scientific and medical literature. Examples of such concepts include: trigger points, motor points, the autonomic nervous system, and neuropeptides such as endorphins. Disease categories are typically those of modern pathophysiology. The different models of practice within and between countries are usually not congruent with each other; while they are superficially similar in that they use, for example, traditional or modern scientific explanations, these explanatory models are often contradictory and often quite distinct.

The historical literature also describes treatment approaches in a variety of different ways. There are treatments based on an assessment of the patient in terms of traditionally conceived ideas of physiology (*jing-luo*, *zang-fu*, *yin-yang*, *qi*, etc.), with treatment aimed at correcting those perceived problems. These are sometimes called *zhi ben*, (root treatment) approaches, in contradistinction to the *zhi biao* (branch treatment) approaches, which target relief of symptoms. Sometimes the *zhi ben* and *zhi biao* treatment approaches were combined, and at other times were applied separately. In each approach there have been many models, depending upon the author and the historical period. Table 3.2 gives examples of historical and modern sources for *zhi ben* and *zhi biao* approaches.

Table 3.2 Examples of root/symptom treatment approaches

	Historical examples	Modern examples
Zhi ben root treatment	*Huang Di Nei Jing Su Wen* (*c.* 200 BC) (see Liao, 1992) Mi (282) (see Yang and Chace, 1994)	Fukushima (1991) Shudo (1990) Wiseman (1985)
Zhi biao symptom control treatment	*Huang Di Nei Jing Su Wen* (*c.* 200 BC (see Liao, 1992) Mi (282) (see Yang and Chace, 1994)	Serizawa and Kusumi (1988) So (1987) Ulett (1992)
Zhi ben and *zhi biao* treatment	Mi (282) (see Yang and Chace, 1994) Yang Ji-zhou (1601) (see Yang and Liu, 1994)	Manaka, Itaya and Birch (1995) Soulie de Morant (1994)

Table 3.3 gives examples from the five countries listed in Table 3.1 of the varied techniques that are applied by acupuncturists as part of the practice of acupuncture. While not exhaustive, it illustrates the range of methods.

One can clearly see in Tables 3.1–3.3 a broad range of models, methods and treatment approaches. Acupuncture is also practised in many different contexts. In China today it is practised in a number of different ways: i) as part of the first tier of medical care (what began as the practice of the 'barefoot doctors'), including basic Western medicine, paramedical treatments, herbal medicine, acupuncture and massage (Rosenthal, 1987); (ii) as part of the practice of 'traditional medicine' in Western-style hospitals, often combined with herbal medicine or massage (Liu, 1988; Wiseman and Ellis, 1985); (iii) as a specialised method employed independently of other medical techniques (Cheng, 1987); (iv) as an adjunct to Western medical care, for example in surgery (Anon. 1975); and (v) as a recently re-emerged independent method of health care practised outside of mainstream health care (Western or traditional), part of the new market system of China (Zhu, 1993). In Japan, on the other hand, acupuncture is mostly practised in private practice outside of the practice of Western medicine and herbal medicine, but often with massage (Birch, 1989–1991; Nakagawa, 1987; Sonoda, 1988). Acupuncture, moxibustion and massage are each licensed separately (Birch, 1989–1991; Nakagawa, 1987; Sonoda, 1988), with many practising each, and some specialising in only one (e.g. Irie, 1980). While some practise acupuncture with herbal medicine, for legal reasons it is mostly practised independently of herbal medicine (Birch, 1989–1991). It is also practised in a large number of hospitals, and is thus practised as a technique partially integrated into standard care. Other countries manifest further diversity, where it is integrated with other traditional medicines such as herbal medicine (Maciocia, 1994), or homoeopathy (Kenyon, 1983, 1985; Voll, 1975), or utilised as a speciality technique within Western medical clinics such as pain clinics (Chapman and Gunn, 1990;

Table 3.3 Examples of the diverse methods employed in acupuncture

	China	Japan	France	USA	UK
Needling with *de qi* type stimulation (sensations of 'soreness' numbness, heaviness, distension' (Cheng, 1987, p. 326) or 'sharp, pulling, electric, tingling, heavy, pulsing, spreading, pricking, aching or hot' (Vincent *et al.*, 1989)	Anon. (1980) Cheng (1987) O'Connor and Bensky (1981) So (1987)	Zheng (1991)	Auteroche et al. (1992) Requena (1986) Soulie de Morant (1994)	Anon. (1980) Cheng (1987) O'Connor and Bensky (1981)	Maciocia (1994)
Needling with no *de qi* type stimulation	Zhang (1979)	Akabane (1986a, b) Fukushima (1991) Manaka, Itaya and Birch (1995) Shudo (1990)		Fukushima (1991) Manaka, Itaya and Birch (1995) Shudo (1990)	
Shallow needling	Bischko (1986, p. 29)	Akabane (1986a) Fukushima (1991) Shudo (1990)	Soulie de Morant (1994)	Birch and Ida (in press) Shudo (1990)	
Non-inserted needling		Birch and Ida (in press) Fukushima (1991) Mori and Yoneyama (1983)		Birch and Ida (in press) Fukushima (1991)	
Needling to stimulate nerve structures	O'Connor and Bensky (1981, p. 467–9)	Serizawa and Kusumi (1988)		Ulett (1992)	Baldry (1989)
Electroacupuncture	Cheng (1987) O'Connor and Bensky (1981)	Shimizu (1986)	Mussat (1972)	Ulett (1992)	Baldry (1989)
Tiny electrical stimulation		Manaka, Itaya and Birch (1995)		Manaka, Itaya and Birch (1995) Matsumoto and Birch (1988)	
Two-metal contact or magnets	Chen (1979)	Nagatomo (1976)		Matsumoto and Birch (1986)	

Table 3.3 (*continued*)

	China	Japan	France	USA	UK
Moxibustion	Anon. (1980) Cheng (1987) O'Connor and Bensky (1981) So (1987)	Akabane (1986b) Birch and Ida (in press) Irie (1980) Manaka, Itaya and Birch (1995)	Auteroche *et al.* (1992) Soulie de Morant (1994)	Birch and Ida (in press) Ellis, Wiseman and Boss (1988)	
Cupping	Cheng (1987) O'Connor and Bensky (1981) Wang and Ren (1985)	Meguro (1991)	Auteroche *et al.* (1992)	Birch and Ida (in press)	
Bloodletting	Wang and Ren (1985)	Maruyama and Kudo (1982)	Auteroche *et al.* (1992)	O'Connor and Bensky (1981)	
Surgical applications	Anon. (1975) O'Connor and Bensky (1981)				

Gaupp, Flinn and Weddige, 1989) and drug abuse treatment centres (Brumbaugh, 1993; Culliton and Kiresuk, 1996). There is clearly no one approach to the practice of acupuncture. It is practised as an independent medical system, a method couched within other systems or as a discrete set of techniques integrated into other models of health care. In short, acupuncture is a multimodal system of healing with multiple competing explanatory models delivered within or outside of multiple health care delivery systems.

CONTEMPORARY ACCOUNTS OF ACUPUNCTURE FAIL TO TAKE ACCOUNT OF ITS DIVERSITY

Despite the ready availability of evidence of diversity in acupuncture, most commentators make more limited descriptions which they then use as if they applied to the whole field. This problem is further compounded when these more limited descriptions are stated in a way that implies that other descriptions or methods are wrong or ineffective. For example, many modern Chinese influenced texts state that for acupuncture to be effective, '*de qi* ' must be obtained at every site needled (Anon. 1980; Cheng, 1987); 'in the process of acupuncture, no matter what manipulation it is, the arrival of *qi* <u>must</u> be achieved. . . . When the patient feels soreness, numbness, heaviness and distension around the point, or their transmission upward and downward along the meridians, it is a sign of the arrival of *qi* (Cheng 1987, p. 326). Authors from other traditions insist that this is not necessary (Fukushima, 1991; Manaka, Itaya and Birch, 1995; Shudo, 1990), or interpret the sensations of '*de qi* ' quite differently (Manaka, Itaya and Birch, 1995; Shudo, 1990). Authors writing about the modern Chinese system, 'traditional Chinese medicine' (TCM), have usually followed the contra-indication that moxibustion should not be used in febrile conditions or when the patient is hot (Anon. 1980; Cheng, 1987; O'Connor, 1981), yet moxibustion specialists in Japan routinely use moxa for precisely those conditions (Irie, 1980), and recent scientific research in China has suggested that moxa is effective for febrile conditions (Tian and Wang, 1987; Wang, Tian and Li, 1987). Some authors claim that for acupuncture to be practised correctly it must be practised according to the principles of Chinese medicine, and that treatments must be made accordingly (Bensoussan, 1991; Diebschlag 1993; Maciocia, 1993): 'In order to get the most out of acupuncture treatment, symptoms must be interpreted according to the theoretical framework of traditional Chinese medicine and treated accordingly' (Diebschlag, 1993); 'A good understanding of TCM is necessary in order to be able to treat pain successfully with acupuncture' (Bensoussan, 1991, p. 21); This model of Chinese medicine is implied to cover all 'traditionally' based models (see Maciocia, 1989, p. ix) yet refers only to the current model from China or a Westernised version of it. Despite the absence of comparative studies and hence any data to support this claim, such authors *de facto* imply that to practise other than the models they describe is wrong. Some who practise acupuncture with herbal medicine following a model that developed in China in the 1960s and 1970s insist that acupuncture has to be practised with herbal medicine to constitute a valid treatment. For example, herbal medicine is a necessary component of the acupuncture licence in California. The fact that this model of practice has already changed to one of specialised practices in China (Ergil, 1993, 1994a, 1994b), and the fact that acupuncture is routinely practised separately from herbal medicine in, for example Japan, appears to be either unknown or simply ignored.

Some authors, in an effort to make their descriptions of acupuncture more palatable to their audience, have added, omitted or distorted key aspects of what they describe. Inaccurate and fanciful descriptions of the history of acupuncture can be found which are intended to help legitimise and popularise a particular 'traditional' model of practice. The preface of a popular text (Maciocia, 1989, p. vii) describes how a peasant woman in 154 BC went for acupuncture (which was not available to peasants at that time (Unschuld, 1985, p. 93), was diagnosed with a condition that would not be described for many centuries (Morohashi, 1976) and was treated by a method that would not be described for that condition for almost two millennia (Cui and Zhang,

1989). The author then attempts to tie this fanciful history to the modern practice of TCM acupuncture as an example of the historical origins of that modern practice, and hence a validation and justification of it. Of these kinds of misrepresentation, Unschuld comments 'Chinese publications, especially those of the last three or four decades, as well as virtually all Western authors promoting traditional Chinese medicine as an alternative to Western medicine, have depicted traditional Chinese medicine, in contrast to historical evidence, as a coherent system of thought, basically unchanged since antiquity' (Unschuld, 1992, p. 54.) On the other hand, distorted traditional descriptions that are intended to ridicule the models from which they supposedly derive can also be found. Melzack, Stillwell and Fox (1977) describe the acupuncture points as being 'associated with an ancient conceptual but anatomically non-existent system of meridians which carry Yin (spirits) and Yang (blood)'. This is a very strange distortion of the language and models of the channels (meridians) and their points, and curiously, is not referenced to any source. Furthermore, it states the authors' untested opinions (that the channels are non-existent), as though those opinions were proven facts. There are examples where modern twentieth-century concepts have been added to 'traditional' models of practice that have no legitimate relationship to that 'tradition'. Pachuta, in a seemingly academic account of acupuncture (Pachuta, 1989, p. 67), makes the following remarkable statement: 'In the Eastern systems, centeredness and wholeness of the practitioner are crucial, and love is essential to the cure.' It is difficult to imagine how to translate these concepts into Chinese, and where in the Chinese literature one might find such concepts. The term 'love', for example, is not only absent in the technical vocabulary of Chinese medicine and acupuncture (Wiseman and Boss, 1990), but its equivalent Chinese term the character 'ai ' (Matthews, 1979, p. 2) can be found only once in the classic acupuncture texts of the *Nei Jing*, the *Huang Di Nei Jing Su Wen* and *Ling Shu* (Kitasato, 1979, 1982). The term 'love' is hardly a 'crucial' or 'essential' concept in acupuncture. This overlay of 1960s Western idealism is not uncommon. There are also examples where significant aspects of the practice of acupuncture are sometimes omitted by particular proponents, for example the model of practice called 'traditional acupuncture' teaches that it is incorrect to treat the symptoms, rather one should focus on the 'causative factor' (CF) (Worsley, 1973, p. 3). This view excludes the huge body of literature from hundreds of texts over two millennia which describe various treatment strategies for relieving specific symptoms. Unschuld has discussed how these distortions have crept into the modern Western literature on acupuncture: 'it is quite inappropriate to select one single facet or approach one single level and call this facet or level "Chinese medicine" – as is done so often today – simply because here we find what many are searching for, an alternative to current Western medicine.' (Unschuld, 1987; see also Unschuld, 1992).

Many more examples could be added to illustrate how proponents of a particular school promote a limited or incorrect idea and then attempt to generalise it to the whole field. It is of course to be expected that a medical system as old and broadly practised as acupuncture should have a widely discrepant corpus of literature. It is also to be expected that a system of medicine from non-Western cultures couched in the language and concepts native to those cultures, would suffer distortion through problems with translation (Unschuld, 1989; Wiseman, 1995; Wiseman and Boss, 1990), and the availability of trans-lated materials (Birch and Tsutani, 1996; Unschuld, 1989, p. ix). While these issues pose problems for the average practitioner, the difficulties they pose for the scientist wishing to research acupuncture are even more significant. Unfor-tunately, many of these issues have not emerged before in the scientific investi-gation of acupuncture. This has both undermined the validity of some research efforts and has rendered many studies difficult to interpret. Central to much of this debate is an argument about the nature of the 'paradigm' of acupuncture and whether acupuncture is 'holistic' or not, and thus whether it must be applied and tested according to 'traditional' principles.

ACUPUNCTURE AS HOLISTIC MEDICINE?

Though there are many claims that acupuncture is 'holistic', we saw in Table 3.1 some modern models of practice that are clearly not 'holistic' (Baldry, 1989; Debata, 1990; Ulett, 1992). Though this is discussed briefly elsewhere (Birch, 1995a; Unschuld, 1987, 1992), it is useful to examine the nature of the 'paradigm' of acupuncture and claims that acupuncture is a form of holistic medicine.

It is assumed by many authors that the underlying 'paradigms' of acupunc-ture and Western (or bio)-medicine are quite different (Cassidy, 1995; Rubik, 1995), and that acupuncture is 'holistic' (Beinfield and Korngold, 1991; Cassidy, 1995; Hammer, 1990; Kaptchuk, 1983; World Health Organization, 1995). 'The Chinese method is thus holistic' (Kaptchuk, 1983, p. 7); 'Acupunc-ture was developed as a branch of traditional Chinese medicine on the basis of oriental philosophy which takes a holistic approach to regulating the balance of the human body' (World Health Organization, 1995). The term 'holistic' is rarely defined clearly in the Western acupuncture literature. A holistic model can be one in which the whole person is taken into account (see e.g. Kaptchuk, 1983, p. 7). A holistic model can also be one where the theoretical nature of the body posits a total interaction of all parts with each other so that none exists or functions independently of the rest (this model is articulated in Needham, 1956; Rubik, 1995). A further viewpoint on holism posits a more ideological position (see Birch, 1995a; Capra, 1982; Dossey 1982; Foss and Rothenberg, 1987). It is argued that Western science and medicine are based on a Cartesian philosophy that perceives a dualism of body and mind, which are considered as though they were separate entities. In this model the reductionist approach is important: to understand how something works, one needs to examine the smaller components that make up that thing; the big picture is simply the sum of its parts. This model further supposes a simple cause and effect relationship whereby the actions of particular things (effects) are the result of prior events or actions (causes). The 'holistic' model supposes a different set of assumptions: the mind and body constitute an inseparable whole, completely interrelated, in denial of Cartesian dualism; the whole is greater than the sum of its parts, in opposition to the reductionist model; and all things interact with each other, so there is no simple cause and effect relationship between one event and another.

There are many philosophical and ideological arguments about these two basic approaches (Birch, 1995a; Capra, 1982; Dossey, 1982; Foss and Rothenberg, 1987). What is important here is that many Western authors see in the traditional explanations of acupuncture the basis for a more holistic model of the body and system of medical practice (e.g. Connelly, 1979; Jarrett, 1995; Kaptchuk, 1983; Rubik, 1995). It is posited that in the traditional model of acupuncture, the mind and body were never discussed separately – seen in the schools of thought that talk about the 'body-mind' or 'body-mind-spirit' (e.g. Connelly, 1979; Jarrett, 1995; Larre, Schatz and Rochat de la Vallee, 1986; Maciocia, 1989; Pachuta, 1989). It is also posited that the traditional models are non-reductionist and acausal, describing how all things interact all the time with all other things and how the whole is greater than the sum of its parts (e.g. Beinfield and Korngold, 1991; Connelly, 1979; Rubik, 1995).

While it is true that there are models, concepts and theories within the traditional explanatory models of acupuncture that are 'holistic', it is also true that there are many important and not insignificant examples of models, concepts and theories that are clearly not 'holistic'. Unschuld (1987, 1992) and Chiu (1986) detail many historical examples that clearly argue against universal statements of 'holism' in the traditional explanatory models. For example, just as in modern Western medicine, many treatment strategies focus on removing or killing pathological agents that have penetrated the body from the outside (bacteria, viruses), so too does Chinese medicine use treatment strategies that focus on removing or doing battle with pathological agents that have penetrated the body from the outside (wind, cold, damp) (Unschuld, 1987, 1992). This stands in stark contrast to the purely holistic models of Chinese medicine put forward by many modern proponents. The traditional model was essentially polyparadigmatic. Unschuld clearly illustrates the existence of multiple competing explanatory models and concepts in the historical and modern literature on acupuncture. 'Holistic' models and concepts are routinely set out alongside or in opposition to non-holistic (what Unschuld has called 'ontological') models or concepts (Unschuld, 1987, 1992). The picture is far more complex than many Western authors have tried to portray: 'the alleged antagonism between a holistic-individualistic Chinese medicine and an ontological–localistic Western medicine is a drastic and misleading historical simplification of both traditions. The issue is far more complex than is usually thought.' (Unschuld, 1992, p. 57). Thus, while it is not correct to argue an across-the-board 'holism' for the traditional models of acupuncture and related systems, it is also clear that many aspects of these models are 'holistic'.

RESEARCH IMPLICATIONS OF DIVERSITY IN ACUPUNCTURE

There are a number of ramifications to these complex multi-tiered theoretical perspectives within the traditional explanatory models. How does one decide which system of acupuncture to follow and test? How does one generalise from the findings of a study testing one of these models or methods to other models or methods? What does the researcher need to look for in a particular description of practice in order to judge the accuracy of what is described?

(1) It is evident that the claim that acupuncture is 'holistic' is problematic, especially when attempting to generalise across the whole field. For example, the insistence that all clinical trials of acupuncture must adhere to testing the 'holistic' nature of acupuncture – in other words that treatments must be based upon traditional (holistic) diagnostic assessments (Bensoussan, 1991; Diebschlag, 1993; Jarrett, 1995; Maciocia 1993) – is not valid. A particular model of practice may be traditional (holistic), but not all models are. Thus different research models may be needed depending on the treatment model tested. This still leaves the problem of how one decides which model of practice to test.

(2) Many authors claim a distinct dichotomy between the 'holistic' integrated models of acupuncture (or Eastern medicine) and the fractured scientific models that underlie biomedical practice and research (or Western medicine) (Beinfield and Korngold, 1991; Jarrett, 1995; Rubik, 1995). Not only does this describe the models underlying acupuncture simplistically and inaccurately (Unschuld, 1987, 1992), it also misrepresents the complex nature of Western medicine, which also has emerging 'holistic' aspects (Foss and Rothenberg, (1987).

Some proponents of this dichotomy argue that it is therefore not possible to use scientific methods, tools and technologies to investigate acupuncture without violating and thus diminishing it (Jarrett, 1995). While it is possible that scientific methods, tools and technologies can be misused in the study of acupuncture, it is not a logical necessity that this will inevitably occur. In any scientific study, investigators must proceed cautiously and become as familiar as possible with the subject under study before designing experiments. To date, failure to do this has been one of the primary shortcoming of scientific investigations of acupuncture. Many investigators appear to have been inadequately informed about the complex nature and details of the practice of acupuncture (for clinical trial examples, see Birch (1995b, 1997)). Birch and Tsutani suggested that problems in the availability of reliable published literature contributed to this inadequacy (Birch and Tsutani, 1996). Many investigators also appear to have taken what proponents have said at face value without questioning it. Unfortunately, as we have seen above, proponents typically describe very limited models. Investigators thus run the risk of investigating things that may be inaccurate, and, in particular, that cannot be generalised. Examples can be found in the clinical trial literature, where inadequate knowledge of the practice of acupuncture has fostered assumptions about what constitutes an adequate treatment, and thus what should be an appropriate control treatment in clinical trials of acupuncture (see Birch, 1995b, 1997). Faulty assumptions about what constitutes the 'real' or 'test' acupuncture treatment usually lead to very poorly conceived notions of what should constitute the 'sham', 'placebo' or 'control' needle treatment. This has undermined many acupuncture trials for the following reasons: (a) what most would consider to be an inadequate treatment is administered as the 'real' or 'test' treatment (e.g. Edelist and Gross, 1976; see Coan *et al.*, 1980); (b) inappropriate treatment is administered as the 'sham', 'placebo' or 'control' treatment where an inactive or placebo treatment is believed to have been applied but instead a very active treatment has been applied (e.g. Wyon *et al.*, 1995; see Birch, 1997); (c) sample size is often inadequate, primarily because of assumptions about the nature of the control treatment.

(3) Establishing 'model fit' and selecting appropriate research methods (Jonas, 1995) is very important in scientific studies of acupuncture. But much greater care needs to be given to this issue than we have seen so far. We must be very careful about any assumptions we make about the nature of the models and we should be willing to utilise a broad range of research methods. For example, if we accept that a particular method of practice we wish to test in a clinical trial is 'holistic', how should we modify the way the study is done, compared with testing a model of practice that we do not consider 'holistic'?

If we test a model that is clearly not 'holistic' in approach, does this let us off the hook? If we assume that 'holistic' models of the body are wrong and focus only on measuring specific outcomes, the fact that we do not attempt to measure more general whole system outcomes could mean that we miss collecting important data. But do we know if general whole system changes occur whether an individualised, more 'holistic' treatment is administered or not?

(4) It should be recognised that there are probably significant limitations in how far the results from a particular study can be generalised, and that therefore care should be taken not to generalise too much. For example, almost all the research validating the opioid peptide models of acupuncture is based on the use of electrical stimulation with needles, especially on animals. The

remainder is based on the use of '*de qi*' type needling. There appears to be no research that has examined other needle techniques to see if the same or similar mechanisms are activated, yet authors often generalise the opioid model across the field. Interestingly this often transpires by a kind of reverse logic: since only electroacupuncture techniques have been clearly shown to activate the opioid peptide mechanisms, then other techniques do not constitute 'real' acupuncture (Ulett 1992), and can thus be used as needle controls in clinical trials (Wyon *et al.*, 1995).

To increase the generalisability of results, it will be necessary to work out some method that allows broader generalisations. Many models or methods need to be experimentally examined and compared. In the design of a study, a neutral treatment approach could be selected that is based on finding significant agreement among a number of diverse sources, as suggested in the BRITS method (Birch, 1995b).

When writing up results from a study, care must be taken to describe accurately the history and nature of acupuncture. One should avoid describing a particular model of practice as though it were reflective of all models. Being careful to cite more reliable sources is important. When citing sources that do not contain the essential ingredients necessary to any good text, it is important to be aware of their limitations. If a text claims to be a translation, it should clearly reference or describe the glossary or dictionary used for that translation. If the text claims to describe a 'traditional' model of practice, it should have adequate referencing of 'traditional' sources. Also beware of excessive use of referencing of secondary sources rather than primary sources. The more secondary sources that are used, the greater the possibility of error.

Clinical trials of particular therapeutic agents, such as pharmaceutical drugs, or therapeutic interventions, such as physical therapy, are not used to argue that 'Western medicine' is of benefit or is not of benefit based upon the results found; rather they are used to conclude that that particular intervention is or is not of benefit. So too in the evaluation of acupuncture, the conclusions from a study testing auricular needling, surface electrical stimulation, electroacupuncture, standard TCM or other methods of acupuncture should not conclude that 'acupuncture' is or is not of benefit; rather one should conclude that that specific acupuncture intervention is or is not of benefit. It is important to be as specific as possible, but many studies have not done so (see Hackett, Seddan and Kaminski, 1988; Ter Riet, Kleijnen and Knipschild, 1990). This not only gives a fairer representation for acupuncture, but also informs acupuncture practitioners, researchers and policy makers about what parts of the field have been shown to be of benefit or not of benefit.

(5) When a researcher consults an acupuncturist, if that person insists that the treatment must be done according to a particular set of principles (e.g. according to the principles of 'traditional Chinese medicine'), or done a certain

way ('*de qi*' must be achieved at every point, electrical stimulation must be applied, etc.), it is good to question this and request that the acupuncturist provide evidence to support what they claim. If there are issues that cannot be resolved, even after consulting other acupuncturists, it may be necessary to consult outside experts (linguists, sinologists, medical historians, etc.). Few acupuncture practitioners can answer technical academic questions or are familiar enough with the issues involved in clinical trial designs. The investigation of acupuncture is likely to need a multidisciplinary approach. The skills of scholars, linguists, basic science researchers, clinical researchers and acupuncture practitioners may need to be invoked in varying degrees in many studies. Unfortunately most research teams have not been so well represented.

CONCLUSION

Many claims about the nature, history, scope, scientific basis and practice of acupuncture appear to be hard to generalise. Acupuncture is a set of therapeutic interventions consisting of multiple methods and utilising a range of diverse explanatory models. However, few practising or writing about acupuncture seem aware of this diversity and its implications; they make claims about acupuncture that are inaccurate or limited or cannot be generalised as intended.

This essay has explored the diversity of acupuncture and discussed examples from the popular, clinical and scientific literature of claims that are inconsistent with that diversity or inconsistent with established facts. Implications, especially for the scientific researcher, were discussed, with potential solutions suggested for a number of critical issues.

Acupuncture is a complex multifaceted field that requires more thorough consideration and more extensive exploration than is usually found in the popular and professional literature about it. If it is to be more thoroughly explored by scientists and other researchers, these issues will need much more attention than they have previously received.

REFERENCES

Akabane, K. (1986a) *Hinaishin Ho* (Intradermal Needle Method), 12th edn, Ido no Nippon Company, Yokosuka.
Akabane K. (1986b) *Kyutoshin Ho* (Moxa on the Handle of the Needle Method), 6th edn, Ido no Nippon Company, Yokosuka.
Anon. (1975) *Acupuncture Anesthesia*, Geographic Health Studies Program, NIH.
Anon. (1980) *Essentials of Chinese Acupuncture*, Foreign Languages Press, Beijing.
Auteroche, B., Gervais, G., Auteroche, M., *et al.*, (1992) *Acupuncture and Moxibustion: A Guide to Clinical Practice*, Churchill Livingstone, Edinburgh.
Baldry, P.E. (1989) *Acupuncture, Trigger Points and Musculoskeletal Pain*, Churchill Livingstone, Edinburgh.

Beinfield, H. and Korngold, E. (1991) *Between Heaven and Earth*, Ballantine Books, New York.

Bensoussan, A. (1991) *The Vital Meridian*, Churchill Livingstone, Edinburgh.

Birch, S. (1989–1991) Acupuncture in Japan; an introductory survey. *Review*, Part 1, **6**, 12–13; Part 2, **7**, 16–20; Part 3, **8**, 21–6; Part 4, **9**, 28–31; 39–42.

Birch, S. (1995a) Introduction, in *Chasing the Dragon's Tail* (eds Y. Manaka, K. Itaya, S. Birch), Paradigm Publications, Brookline, MA.

Birch, S. (1995b) Testing the clinical specificity of needle sites in controlled clinical trials of acupuncture: Part 1 – the importance of validating the 'relevance' of 'true' or 'active' points and 'irrelevance' of 'control' or 'less-active' points – proposal for a justification method, in *Proceedings of the Second Symposium of the Society for Acupuncture Research*, Society for Acupuncture Research, Washington, DC, pp. 274–94.

Birch, S. (1995c) Letter to the editor. *Complementary Therapies in Medicine*, **3**(1), 57.

Birch, S. (1997) Issues to consider in determining an adequate treatment in a clinical trial of acupuncture. *Complementary Therapies in Medicine*, **5**, 8–12.

Birch, S. and Felt, R. (in press) *Understanding Acupuncture*, Churchill Livingstone, Edinburgh.

Birch, S. and Ida, J. (in press) *Japanese Acupuncture: A Clinical Guide*, Paradigm Publications, Brookline, MA.

Birch, S. and Tsutani, K. (1996) A bibliometrical study of English-language materials on acupuncture. *Complementary Therapies in Medicine*, **4**, 172–9.

Bischko, J. (1986) *Intermediate Acupuncture* volume 2, Karl F. Haug Publishers, Heidelberg.

Brumbaugh, A. (1993) Acupuncture: new perspectives in chemical dependency treatment. *Journal of Substance Abuse Treatment*, **10**, 35–43.

Capra, F. (1982) *The Turning Point*, Bantam Books, New York.

Cassidy, C.M. (1994) Ethnography of an acupuncture training program. Paper presented at the American Anthropological Association meeting in Atlanta.

Cassidy, C.M. (1995) Social science theory and methods in the study of alternative and complementary medicine. *Journal of Alternative and Complementary Medicine* **1**(1), 19–40.

Chapman C.R. and Gunn, C.C. (1990) Acupuncture, in *The Management of Pain*. Volume 1, 2nd edn (ed. J.J. Bonica), Lea & Febiger, Philadelphia, 1805–21.

Chen Zhi (1979); *Ci Liao Fa* (Magnet Treatment Methods), Science & Technology Publishing Company, Hunan.

Cheng, X.N. (1987) *Chinese Acupuncture and Moxibustion*, Foreign Languages Press, Beijing.

Chiu, M.L. (1986) Mind, body, and illness in a Chinese medical tradition. PhD thesis, Harvard University, Cambridge, MA.

Connelly, D. (1979) *Traditional Acupuncture: The Law of the Five Elements*, The Centre for Traditional Acupuncture, Columbia, MD.

Cui Jin and Zhang Guang-qi (1989) A survey for thirty years clinical application of cupping. *Journal of Traditional Chinese Medicine*, **9**(2), 151–4.

Culliton, P.D. and Kiresuk, T.J. (1994) Overview of substance abuse acupuncture treatment research. *Journal of Alternative and Complementary Medicine*, **2**(1), 149–59.

Debata, A. (1990) *Kaigyo Shinkyushi no tameno Shinsatsuho to Chiryoho* (Diagnosis and Treatment of Sciatica for the Private Practitioner Acupuncturist), 4th edn Ido no Nippon Sha, Yokosuka.

Diebschlag, F. (1993) Placebo acupuncture. *European Journal of Oriental Medicine*, **1**(2), 12–17.

Dossey, L. (1982) *Space, Time and Medicine*, Shambhala Publications, Boulder.

Edelist, G. and Gross, A.E. (1976) Treatment of low back pain with acupuncture. *Canadian Anaesthesiologists Society Journal*, **23**(3), 303–6.

Ellis, A., Wiseman, N. and Boss, K. (1988) *Fundamentals of Chinese Acupuncture*, Paradigm Publications, Brookline, MA.

Ergil, M.C. (1993) Letter to the editor. *Journal of the Acupuncture Society of New York*, **1–3**, 23–6.

Ergil, M.C. (1994a) Medical education in China. *CCAOM News*, **1**(1), 3–5.

Ergil, M.C. (1994b) Chinese medicine in China: education and learning strategies. Paper presented at Association for Asian Studies Annual Meeting, Boston.

Foss, L. and Rothenberg, K. (1987) *The Second Medical Revolution*, Shambhala Publications, Boston.

Fukushima, K. (1991) *Meridian Therapy*, Toyo Hari Medical Association Tokyo.

Gaupp, L.A., Flinn, D.E. and Weddige, R.L. (1989) Adjunctive treatment techniques, in *Handbook of Chronic Pain Management* (ed. C.D. Tollison), Williams & Wilkins, Baltimore pp. 174–6.

Hackett, G.I., Seddon, D. and Kaminski, D. (1988) Electroacupuncture compared with paracetamol for acute low back pain. *The Practitioner*, **232**, 163–4.

Hammer, L. (1990) *Dragon Rises Red Bird Flies*, Station Hill Press, Barrytown, NY.

Helms, J.M. (1995) *Acupuncture Energetics: A Clinical Approach for Physicians*, Medical Acupuncture Publishers, Berkeley.

Huang Di Nei Jing Su Wen (The Yellow Emperor's Classic of Internal Medicine) (*c*. 200 BC). For a translation of chapter 41, see Liao (1992).

Irie, S. (1980) *Fukaya Kyu Ho* (Fukaya's Moxa Method), Shizensha Tokyo.

Jarrett, L. (1995) Letter to the editor. *Journal of the Acupuncture Society of New York*, **2**(1), 6–11.

Jonas, W.B. (1995) Balancing quality research in acupuncture: matching methodology with goals and materials, in *Proceedings of the Second Symposium of the Society for Acupuncture Research*, Society for Acupuncture Research, Washington, DC, pp. 212–29.

Kaptchuk, T.J. (1983) *The Web that Has No Weaver*, Congdon and Weed, New York.

Kenyon, J.N. (1983) *Modern Techniques of Acupuncture*, volume 1, Thorsons Publishing Group, Wellingborough.

Kenyon, J.N. (1985) *Modern Techniques of Acupuncture*, volume 3. Thorsons Publishing Group, Wellingborough.

Kitasato kenkyujo huzoku toyoigaku sogokenkyujo rinsho koten kenkyuhan (1979) *Reisu Rinsho Sakuinshu*, the Suwen Clinical Index, Kokusho Kankokai, Tokyo.

Kitasato kenkyujo huzoku toyoigaku sogokenkyujo rinsho koten kenkyuhan (1982) *Somon Rinsho Sakuinshu*, the Lingshu Clinical Index, Kokusho Kankokai, Tokyo.

Larre, C., Schatz, J. and Rochat de la Vallee, E. (1986) *Survey of Traditional Chinese Medicine*, l'Institute Ricci, Paris.

Liao, S.J. (1992) Acupuncture for low back pain in *Huang Di Nei Jing Su Wen*. *Acupuncture and Electrotherapeutics Research International Journal*, **17**, 249–58.

Liao, S.J., Lee, M.H.M. and Ng L.K. (1994) *Principles and Practice of Contemporary Acupuncture*, Marcel Dekker, New York.

Liu Bing-quan (1988) *Optimum Time for Acupuncture*, Shandong Science & Technology Press, Jinan.

Liu Yan-chi (1988) *The Essential Book of Traditional Chinese Medicine*, Columbia University Press, New York.

Lu, G.D. and Needham, J. (1980) *Celestial Lancets*, Cambridge University Press Cambridge.

Maciocia, G. (1989) *Foundations of Chinese Medicine*, Churchill Livingstone, Edinburgh.

Maciocia, G. (1993) Letter to the editor. *Complementary Therapies in Medicine* 1(4), 221–2.

Maciocia, G. (1994) *The Practice of Chinese Medicine*, Churchill Livingstone, Edinburgh.

Manaka, Y., Itaya K. and Birch, S. (1995) *Chasing the Dragon's Tail*, Paradigm Publications Brookline, MA.

Mann, F. (1974) *Treatment of Disease by Acupuncture*, William Heinemann Medical Books, London.

Maruyama, M. and Kudo K. (1982) *Shinpan Shiraku Ryoho* (Bloodletting Therapy), Seki Bundo Publishing Company, Tokyo.

Matsumoto, K. and Birch S. (1986) *Extraordinary Vessels*, Paradigm Publications, Brookline, MA.

Matsumoto, K. and Birch, S. (1988) *Hara Diagnosis: Reflections on the Sea*, Paradigm Publications, Brookline, MA.

Matthews Chinese–English Dictionary (1979). Harvard University Press, Cambridge, MA.

Meguro, A. (1991) *Kyukau Ryoho* (Cupping Therapy), 5th edn, Midori Shobo Publishing Company, Tokyo.

Melzack, R. Stillwell, D.M. and Fox, E.J. (1977) Trigger points and acupoints for pain: correlations and implications. *Pain*, **3**, 3–23.

Mi, H.F. (282) *Zhen Jiu Jia Yi Jing* (The Systematic Classic of Acupuncture and Moxibustion). For a translation of the text, see Yang and Chace (1994).

Mori, H. and Yoneyama, H. (1983) *Shonishin Ho* (Acupuncture for Children), Ido no Nippon Sha, Yokosuka.

Morohashi, T. (ed.) (1976) *Daikanwa Jiten* (Morohashi Encyclopedic Dictionary of Chinese), 5th edn, Daishukan Sha, Tokyo.

Mussat, M. (1972) *Physique de l'Acupuncture: Hypotheses et Approches Experimentales* (The Physics of Acupuncture: Hypotheses and Experimental Approaches), Libraire le Francois, Paris.

Nagatomo, T. (1976) *Nagatomo MP Shinkyu Kuowa Hachiju Hachisyu* (Nagatomo's 88 Lectures on Minus–Plus Needle Therapy), Shinkyu Shinkuokai, Kyoto.

Nakagawa, Y. (1987) The present situation for acupuncture and moxibustion clinics and practitioners in Japan. *Ido no Nippon Magazine*, **406**(7), 515, 102–7; **46**(8), 516, 91–5.

Needham, J. (1956) *Science and Civilisation in China*, volume 2, Cambridge University Press, Cambridge.

Nogier, P.F.M. (1983) *From Auriculotherapy to Auriculomedicine*, Maisonneuve, Saint-Ruffine.

O'Connor, J. and Bensky, D. (1981) *Acupuncture: A Comprehensive Text*, Eastland Press, Seattle.

Pachuta, D.M. (1989) Chinese medicine: the law of five elements in *Eastern and Western Approaches to Healing* (eds A.A. Sheikh and K.S. Sheikh), John Wiley & Sons, New York.

Requena, Y. (1986) *Terrains and Pathology in Acupuncture*, Paradigm Publications, Brookline, MA.

Rosenthal, M.M. (1987) *Health Care in the People's Republic of China: Moving Toward Modernization*, Westview Press, Boulder.

Rubik, B. (1995) Can Western science provide a foundation for acupuncture? *Alternative Therapies in Health and Medicine*, **1**(4), 41–7.

Serizawa, K. and Kusumi, M. (1988) *Clinical Acupuncture*, Japan Publications Inc, Tokyo.

Shimizu, K. (1986) Pressure pain points, diagnosis and treatments. *Ido no Nippon Magazine*, **45**(4), 500: 315–24.

Shudo, D. (1990) *Japanese Classical Acupuncture: Introduction to Meridian Therapy*, Eastland Press, Seattle.

So, J.T.Y. (1987) *Treatment of Disease with Acupuncture*, Paradigm Publications, Brookline, MA.

Sonoda, K. (1988) *Health and Illness in Changing Japanese Society*, University of Tokyo Press, Tokyo.

Soulie de Morant, G. (1994) *Chinese Acupuncture*, Paradigm Publications, Brookline, MA.

Suehara, I. (1985) *Genso Keiraku Ho* (Fundamental Meridian Therapy), Onso Shindangaku Kenkyujo Research Institute, Tokyo.

Ter Reit, G., Kleijnen, J. and Knipschild, P. (1990); Acupuncture and chronic pain: a criteria-based meta-analysis. *Journal of Clinical Epidemiology*, **43**(11), 1191–9.

Tian Conghuo and Wang Yin (1987) Clinical and experimental research on the antipyretic effects of moxibustion, in *Selection from Article Abstracts on Acupuncture and Moxibustion*, Association of Acupuncture and Moxibustion, Beijing, 221–2.

Ulett, G. (1992) *Beyond Yin and Yang*, Warren H. Green, St. Louis.

Unschuld, P.U. (1985) *Medicine in China: A History of Ideas*, University of California Press, Berkeley.

Unschuld, P.U. (1987) Traditional Chinese medicine; some historical and epistemological reflections. *Social Science and Medicine*, **24**(12), 1023–9.

Unschuld, P.U. (ed.) (1989) *Approaches to Traditional Chinese Medical Literature*, Kluwer Academic Publishers, Dordrecht.

Unschuld, P.U. (1992) Epistemological issues and changing legitimation: traditional Chinese medicine in the twentieth century in *Paths to Asian Medical Knowledge*, (eds C. Leslie and A. Young), University of California Press, Berkeley.

Vincent, C.A., Richardson, P.H., Black, J.J. and Pither, C.E. (1989) The significance of needle placement site in acupuncture: *Journal of Psychosomatic Research*, **33**(4), 489–96.

Voll, R. (1975) Twenty years of electroacupuncture diagnosis in Germany; a progress report. *American Journal of Acupuncture*, **3**, 7–17.

Wang Feng-yi and Ren Huan-zhao (1985) *Kyugyoku Ryoho (Cupping Therapy)*, (trans. Kaname Asakawa), Toyo Gakujutsu Publishing Company, Ichikawa.

Wang Yin, Tian Conghuo and Li Zhiming (1987) Preliminary observation on the treatment of fever due to the invasion of exogenous pathogenic wind cold with warm moxibustion in *Selections from Article Abstracts on Acupuncture and Moxibustion*, China Association on Acupuncture and Moxibustion, Beijing, p. 220–1.

Wiseman, N. (1995) *English–Chinese, Chinese–English Dictionary of Chinese Medicine*, Hunan Science & Technology Publishers, Hunan.

Wiseman, N. and Ellis, A. (1985) *Fundamentals of Chinese Medicine*, Paradigm Publications, Brookline, MA.

Wiseman, N. and Boss, K. (1990) *Glossary of Chinese Medical Terms and Acupuncture Points*, Paradigm Publications, Brookline, MA.

World Health Organization (1985) The role of traditional medicine in primary health care. WPR/RC36/Technical Discussions/s, World Health Organization, Manila.

World Health Organization (1995) *Guidelines for Clinical Research on Acupuncture*, World Health Organization, Manila.

Worsley, J.R. (1973) *Is Acupuncture for You?* England, College of Traditional Chinese Acupuncture, Leamington Spa.

Wyon, Y., Lindgren, R., Lundeberg, T. and Hammar, M. (1995) Effects of acupuncture on climacteric vasomotor symptoms, quality of life, and urinary excretion of neuropeptides among postmenopausal women. *Menopause: The Journal of the North American Menopause Society*, **2**(1), 3–12.

Yang Ji-zhou (1601) *Zhen Jiu Da Cheng* (Great Compendium of Acupuncture and Moxibustion). For translations of portions of the text, see Matsumoto & Birch (1986), Yang & Liu (1994).

Yang Shou-zhong and Chace, C. (1994) *The Systematic Classic of Acupuncture and Moxibustion*, Blue Poppy Press, Boulder.

Yang Shou-zhong and Liu Feng-ting (1994) *The Divinely Responding Classic*, Blue Poppy Press, Boulder.

Zhang Xin-shu (1979) *Sokkon Shin* (Wrist Ankle Acupuncture) (trans. by Matsutane Sugi), Ido no Nippon sha, Yokokusa.

Zheng Kui-shan (1991) *Sashin demiru Shinkyu Hosha Shugi* (An Illustrated Manual of Acu-moxa Supplementation and Draining Techniques) (trans. Akira Hyodo), Goto School of TCM Research Department, Tokyo.

4 | Homoeopathic therapeutics: many dimensions – or meaningless diversity?

Jeremy Swayne

INTRODUCTION

Medicine is both an academic discipline and, for many of us, a vocation. There is a tension between the intellectual rigour of the one and the intuitive impulse of the other, which can be uncomfortable. At its most extreme this tension becomes polarised as a struggle between the mechanistic and the holistic. This should be a false dichotomy. The mechanistic can be the antithesis of the holistic; but holism, the perception of the whole as being more than the sum of its parts, includes and comprehends the part that is mechanical, and the mechanistic method may be put entirely and essentially at the service of a holistic purpose.

This chapter examines the holistic nature of the vocational impulse in medicine and the enthusiasm that homoeopathy arouses in those who favour a holistic approach. It goes on to discuss the grounds for scepticism that abound in the way that homoeopathic principles and method are applied in practice, and the need to address these through proper academic discipline.

The problem with homoeopathy that I wish to explore is as follows: Homoeopathy has many reasons to justify a claim to be holistic. Its principles and practice require a detailed and integrated study of the many facets of the patient and the illness that make up the whole. But there is extraordinary diversity in the practical application of those principles – so much so that a consistent therapeutic method based on a coherent and unifying rationale is hard to find.

This diversity may reflect some precious truth about human nature and its behaviour in health and illness, but to most critics the reality must appear incoherent and irrational. Many involved in homoeopathy may fear that attempts to impose order and discipline on the development and investigation of its methods will damage its holistic impulse. On the contrary, I believe such discipline is necessary if homeopathy is to fulfil its potential as a form of holistic medicine in its own right and if its holistic and scientific insights are to enhance the evolution of medicine as a whole.

HOLISM IN MEDICAL PRACTICE

If open to the experience, a general practitioner is exposed more than most to the complex panorama of human nature and the interplay between our character and 'constitution', the circumstances of our life, and our health. Experience emphasises the multifactorial and multifaceted nature of illness in individual patients, and encourages understanding and respect for the nature and uniqueness of the 'whole' person.

It also reveals the difference and the relationship between the two tasks of a healing profession, that of controlling and manipulating the mind–body system in order to oppose the disease process or dysfunction, and of enabling and reinforcing the natural resources of mind and body on behalf of the healing process. Unfortunately these are not always easily reconciled and the first may often interfere with the second. This is a tension that a doctor must learn to recognise, understand and manage. Inevitably we discover considerable gaps in our repertoire of skills and insights for achieving both tasks, particularly the latter, and that there is much more to the illness and to the person who is ill than meets even the most enlightened medical eye. The practice of medicine or any branch of health care should be an adventure in holism, and it is this perspective that we may hope will be enhanced by the study of a medical modality that lays particular emphasis on the holistic approach, as homoeopathy and the so-called 'complementary' therapies in general claim to do.

THE HOLISTIC ATTRACTION OF HOMOEOPATHY

There was nothing essentially holistic in the origins of homoeopathy. It was not conceived as a medicine of the whole person but on pragmatic and empirical principles from the observed effects of substances on healthy people and their corresponding benefits when used as medicines for sick people manifesting disorders similar to those effects. Its early triumphs included cholera, an epidemic pathology in which the nature of the individual patient is hardly an issue. Today homoeopathy is still used to good effect on circumscribed, pathological indications, and is gaining respect in veterinary medicine, where the treatment of large populations is common and seldom involves a holistic perspective of the patient.

The simillimum principle (treating like with like, as described above) is not therefore holistic *per se*. Its chief distinction *vis-à-vis* much conventional contemporary Western medicine is its emphasis on enabling the patient's own self-regulatory and healing mechanisms rather than on manipulating and controlling body function and dysfunction. This principle is by inference holistic in as much as it implies an integrated and integrating process of the organism as a whole, and is, of course, central to the philosophy of most nursing care and of professions allied to medicine such as occupational therapy and physiotherapy.

Two other factors contribute to homoeopathy's holistic reputation. One is somewhat esoteric and by no means central to most people's thinking. This is that homoeopathic medicine evokes and strengthens the 'vital force', an energy which sustains all life and all the functions of life, and which is both personal and universal. This concept is primarily metaphysical, although modern understanding of biophysics has made such a fundamental property of life seem more of a physical reality.

The other factor is the emphasis on the individuality of the patient, on the unique experience of the illness in that patient, and on the place and meaning of the illness in the history of the patient. Continuing experimental investigation of the homoeopathic potential of substances through provings (testing in healthy volunteers to elicit their properties), and above all clinical experience, have progressively enriched our understanding of this individuality and our ability to respond to it with the homoeopathic prescription in whose 'likeness' it is reflected. We have no idea how this resonance between the characteristics of the drug and of the ill person comes to be, or how it effects its healing stimulus.

In its fullest form, the homoeopathic approach is comprehensive in its study of the whole experience and manifestation of the illness in individual patients, and of their personal characteristics, life experiences and family background. This attention to detail – the importance of taking seriously all that the patient has to say about the illness, and the belief that it all matters and has meaning – is a healing process in itself. It encourages the patient to see themselves as an integrated whole. It contradicts the sense of fragmentation and depersonalisation which conventional medicine often creates by organising us into separate systems and separate disorders, each with their separate treatments.

This is extremely attractive to any doctor with a holistic intention towards patients. But it also makes it easier to focus attention on those separate elements of the problem that require it, because their separate importance emerges naturally from the whole pattern of which they are a coherent part. These characteristics and the fact that the method appears to get good therapeutic results explain the holistic attraction of homoeopathy.

THE GROUNDS FOR SCEPTICISM

Though arguments for scepticism about homoeopathy have often focused on its biological implausibility, my own worry turns on the bewildering variety of homoeopathic precept and practice. The formal research evidence (Kleijnen, Knipschild and Ter Riet, 1991; Linde *et al.*, 1997; Reilly *et al.*, 1994) is beginning to confer some 'orthodox' intellectual credibility upon the subject, and it is beginning to seem experimentally possible that infinitesimal, ultra-molecular dilutions are biologically active. But even so, is it plausible that this biological property should be the active principle in all the wide diversity of clinical method in which it is allegedly employed?

THE ORIGIN OF DIVERSITY IN HOMOEOPATHY

There is an enormous diversity in the beliefs and practices of homoeopaths. It is arguable that this results from the lack of a mechanistic justification and any means of technical investigation of the biophysical phenomenon its principles suggest. The evolution of homoeopathy since Hahnemann (1755–1843) has paralleled, chronologically, the history of pathology since the time of Pasteur (1822–1895), whose life the successive editions of the *Organon*, Hahnemann's pioneering treatise on homoeopathy, encompassed (1810–1921; see Hahnemann, 1982). Pathology-based medicine has had the advantage of possessing the tools to investigate, validate and develop its early observations and hypotheses in a systematic and convergent manner; each advance in knowledge and method is based on precedent, perhaps contradicting and correcting it, but proceeding coherently from it. The whole history of the development of vaccines and antibiotics from Pasteur onwards exemplifies this feature: the refinement and application of microbiology, epidemiology and pharmacology to the task; the competing claims of different vaccines, in polio for example; the changing status of and indications for particular antibiotics such as sulphonamides, streptomycin, chloramphenicol; the growing problems of multiple resistance in organisms.

By contrast, homoeopathy lacks a coherent and progressing scientific basis. This has allowed a free proliferation of divergent theories composed of metaphysical and empirical observations in varying proportion and relationship. From a philosophical point of view, such diversity is arguably necessary and healthy. But it is extremely confusing for anyone seeking some consistency of clinical method. Further, it can be argued that diversity may not be in the best interests of patients: it is unlikely that all forms of homoeopathy are equally effective; and if they are not, some patients will receive inferior treatment.

DIVERSITY IN HOMOEOPATHIC PHILOSOPHY

In South America, the three most influential teachers of homoeopathy have strikingly different therapeutic ideologies. Two, Paschero and Mazi Elizalde, believe that one fundamental state (miasm) underlies the patient's disposition to and manifestation of illness throughout life. The prescription that correctly reflects this state will be sufficient to their needs throughout life (though practitioners do not claim always to be able to find it). Their views differ, however, in that this fundamental state is attributed by Paschero to environmental factors, and by Masi Elizalde to inherited factors, including disorders of a spiritual nature (Gaier, 1991). By contrast, Eizayaga adopts a more pragmatic approach. His regime focuses first on the primary manifestations of the disease in the patient, those that most urgently invite attention (lesional); then, as these show improvement, on the wider characteristics of the patient (constitutional), and finally on the underlying predisposing or aetiological factors (fundamental). The prescriptions used at each stage may or may not be the same.

DIVERSITY IN PRESCRIBING STRATEGIES

The *Homoeopathica Europa* study groups have identified at least 26 possible types of prescription from which a prescribing strategy may be composed and which are used in different permutations and with different emphases in different countries or by different schools of homoeopathy. At one end of the spectrum are prescriptions with specific applications based on the pathological state or the tissue or organ involved in the disease. At the other are those reflecting the 'essence' of the illness, or rather of the patient with their illness. This may be expressed as a metaphor that embraces both physical and psychological aspects of the disorder and perhaps the circumstances out of which the illness and the characteristics of the individual as a person have arisen. Thus 'coldness' might express the essence of a particular medicine appropriate to the 'essence' of a patient whose emotional upbringing, present psychological state and physical symptoms all reflect the quality of coldness.

In-between are isopathic prescriptions, derived from the causative agent of the disorder; local prescriptions based on the particular characteristics of the presenting problem alone (the precise characteristics of a rash, for example); prescriptions based on the whole pattern of all the patient's problems – the headache, the irritable bowel, and anxiety, perhaps; prescriptions that take account of the constitutional characteristics of the individual; prescriptions based on the pattern of illness in the family history; and so on. Each of these types of prescription have their guiding principles and justification.

DIVERSITY IN USE OF POLYPHARMACY

The number of drugs prescribed during any one phase of a regime also varies. The 'purist' regime will use only one drug, from one source material, moving on to another single prescription only when a new set of prescribing indications, a new 'clinical picture' reveals the need for it. Other regimes will use more than one drug, in sequence or at intervals, related to different aspects or levels of the clinical picture, much as does conventional medicine; a practice known as 'polypharmacy'. Such a regime might include one dose of a prescription based on the patient's constitutional characteristics followed by repeated doses of another prescription reflecting only the features of the local disorder – the joint pain, for example. Other methods use combinations of drugs, complexes, in the form of one dosage, much as a conventional cold cure might contain an analgesic (painkiller) and a decongestant in the same medicine or tablet.

DIVERSITY IN DOSE AND POTENCY

There is also great variety in the use of dosage regimes and potencies. Potencies are medicines of different degrees of dilution produced by a process of which succussion (vigorous shaking) is an essential part. Homoeopathic medicines are sometimes used as 'mother tinctures', that is as undiluted extracts or preparations of the original material, but the dilutions used clinically in accordance with the different perceptions of the illness and different strategies already described range from a series of a few dilutions of one part in ten, to a thousand dilutions of one part in a hundred, or more. The lowest dilutions will contain detectable amounts of the original substance; the higher dilutions will not.

There are principles that govern the choice of low and high potencies, so that a regime may be individually tailored to a patient's condition, but nevertheless there are practitioners who are habitually low potency prescribers and others who habitually prescribe high potencies. In a study of prescribing by members of the UK Faculty of Homoeopathy a wide spectrum of prescribing habits was demonstrated, even though the comparison involved well established practitioners who had been through the same training process (Dempsey and Swayne, 1990). Prescribers B and C in their combined series of 76 cases used the lowest potencies in 65% of them. Prescribers Q and R used the highest potencies in 63% of their 91 cases.

Some prescribers give only one potency at one time, some will give the same drug in a sequence of different potencies, some will give more than one drug in a sequence, each in different potencies. The prescriber giving the 'constitutional' and 'local' prescriptions in sequence in the example above would probably give the former in a higher and the latter in a lower potency.

Depending on the potency, the drug may be repeated at shorter or longer intervals. Usually low potencies are repeated frequently, and higher potencies at greater intervals or only when the progress of the patient requires it. But some prescribers will give high potencies frequently over a period of time even in chronic illness.

DIVERSITY IN MATERIA MEDICA

The uncertain evidence on which much of the data in the materia medica and repertories (drug-symptom cross reference manuals) are based, and the inconsistencies between different repertories can undermine confidence in the prescription derived from them. Comparison of the relevant repertory entries in Kent's and Boericke's repertories (Boericke, 1927; Kent, 1986) the two most commonly used desk references in the UK in recent years, makes it very difficult to discern which medicines are clearly indicated for complaints aggravated by cold dry weather. The presence in one list of some commonly associated with cold wet weather compounds the problem.

THE CONSEQUENCES OF DIVERSITY

This description of the variety and complexity of method in the assessment, interpretation and treatment of patients may seem fantastic to the uninitiated. It has to be said that each permutation of the therapeutic process described here is based on a rationale that has been painstakingly developed by its proponents or by the homoeopathic community as a whole from a great depth of clinical experience and with much deliberation. For example, one method advocates the regular use of low potency remedies based on the physical symptoms in established chronic pathology. In the same situation another method will use one dose of a high potency based perhaps on the 'essence' of the case (see above), with no repetition until the changing clinical picture indicates it. The difference arises from different perceptions of the dynamics of the disease process and of the homoeopathic stimulus, and the interaction between the two.

Each rationale and strategy claims equal success for homoeopathy, though different schools of homoeopathy might identify different goals and outcomes as criteria of success. The low-potency regime might be expected to induce change at the level of the organic lesion alone, whereas the other might expect to achieve a far more comprehensive improvement in the health and well-being of the individual.

The evidence in every country where homeopathy is practised is that patients feel better for it however we do it. This is the worrying thing. This is the ultimate ground of scepticism. If people get better whatever we do, does it actually matter what we do? It is commonly said in conventional medicine that a multiplicity of treatments for any one condition is a measure of how little benefit any of them provide. In homoeopathy, whose patients often choose it because of the limitations of conventional treatments – and claim benefit from it, the problem is slightly different. If all of them work, do any of them really work? Is it that all the various concepts of illness, perceptions of the state of the individual patient, and treatment strategies are valid and lead to a beneficial result in the patient? Or are some concepts, perceptions and strategies valid whereas others are not? Might it be the case that the true activity of the homoeopathic medicine is independent of the different concepts, perceptions and strategies on which the prescription is based, that the medicines do act but on some principle other than those currently described? Or is diversity in homoeopathy evidence that homoeopathic medicines are not active agents but the homoeopathic approach powerfully enhances the placebo effect and that the concepts, perceptions and strategies discussed have a role in enriching this enhanced placebo effect?

DOES DIVERSITY MATTER?

Why should I remain sceptical? And why should I let it bother me? I have nearly twenty years' experience of using homoeopathy, and my 'informed empiricism' – clinical experience and judgement tested against the intellectual disciplines of my medical training – tells me that patients are benefiting from my use of homoeopathy in ways that were not possible before I introduced it to my repertoire of skills. I am able to apply this same informed empiricism and these same intellectual disciplines to the task of studying, testing, criticising, adopting or rejecting the wide variety of therapeutic principles and methods that I have described. I have already alluded to the comforting trickle of hard evidence of the efficacy of these apparently absurd homoeopathic dilutions. Why should I not be content to develop my skills and continue to treat patients as well as I can, and forget my scepticism?

Many holistic thinkers and practitioners might argue that to dissect, analyse and investigate the process is philosophically incompatible with it, and is bound to miss the point. It can be claimed, and rightly I am sure, that the essence of holistic medicine lies in the non-specific effects of the therapeutic transaction, and not in the efficacy of specific agents and specific methods. These non-specific factors include all the factors that are involved in what has come to be described as 'prescribing the drug doctor.' These are of course the milieu of action of the placebo effect itself.

The reason why I keep my scepticism alive and kicking is that it is a stimulating companion to my 'satiable curtiosity'. I am prepared to risk a few intellectual spankings for my curtiosity and scepticism, as did the Elephant's child (Kipling, 1995), in order to investigate the wonder of the world – not to diminish it but to enhance it. This attitude, which I believe to be truly scientific, was expressed beautifully by George Orwell in a broadcast talk on '*The meaning of a poem*' (Orwell, 1970):

> I have tried to analyse this poem as well as I can in a short period, but nothing I have said can explain, or explain away, the pleasure I take in it. That is finally inexplicable, and it is just because it is inexplicable that detailed criticism is worthwhile. Men of science can study the life processes of a flower, or they can split it up into its component elements, but any scientist will tell you that a flower does not become less wonderful, it becomes more wonderful, if you know all about it.

If Orwell was speaking today he might have said 'any *true* scientist', because the distinction between what Schumacher (1995) called science for manipulation and science for understanding, which leads to wisdom, has become more acute since that talk was originally given in 1941. It is science for understanding that Orwell is speaking of and that I would call true science. Be that as it may, it is for these reasons, so clearly expressed by Orwell, that we need to examine rigorously what is going on in homoeopathy.

We need to investigate the efficacy of the specific effects and we need to understand the effectiveness and importance of the non-specific effects. We need to know to what extent the diversity of principle and method that we find in homoeopathy is of metaphysical importance or (ultimately) of pharmacological importance. We need to understand the difference, importance and outcome of the various homoeopathic approaches and the relationship between these and the outcome of the different homoeopathic prescriptions.

We need to investigate the implications of what we observe and what we do both for our understanding of the human organism in health and illness and of the relationship between our organism and the other organisms and inorganic substances that we use in medicinal form as agents of therapeutic change.

This is a huge and amazing field of enquiry, and we need to be courageous, painstaking, intellectually honest and imaginative in asking the appropriate questions. For 'holists' this includes the uncomfortably mechanistic process of formulating testable and refutable hypotheses with which to explore and justify the diversity of precept and practice.

Dissection and analysis – splitting things up into their component elements if done in the right spirit makes things more wonderful. Paying proper attention and respect to the parts is essential to our worship (worth-ship) of the whole. Scepticism and satiable curtiosity are necessary partners in this venture.

REFERENCES

Boericke, W. (1927) *Materia Medica with Repertory*, Boericke & Runyon 1927, Philadelphia.

Dempsey, T. and Swayne, J. (1990) Thinking what we are doing. *British Medical Journal*, **2**, 82–99.

Gaier, H. (1991) Miasma, in *Thorsons Encyclopaedic Dictionary of Homoeopathy*, Thorsons, London.

Hahnemann, S.C. (1982) *Organon of Medicine*, 6th edn, Tarcher, Los Angeles.

Kent, J.T. (1986) *Repertory of the Homoeopathic Materia Medica*, Homoeopathic Book Service, London.

Kipling, R. (1995) *Just So Stories*, Oxford University Press, Oxford.

Kleijnen, J. Knipschild, P. and Ter Riet, G. (1991) Clinical trials of homoeopathy. *British Medical Journal* **302**, 316–23.

Linde, K., Clausuis, N., Ramirez, G., Melchant, D., Eitel, F., Hedges, L.V. and Jonas, W.B. (1997) Are the clinical effects of homoeopathy placebo effects? A meta-analysis of placebo-controlled trials. *Lancet*, **350**(9081), 834–43.

Orwell, G. (1970) The meaning of a poem, in *The Collected Essays, Journalism and Letters of George Orwell*, volume 2, Penguin, Harmondsworth.

Reilly, D. *et al.* (1994) Is the evidence for homoeopathy reproducible? *Lancet* **344**, 1600–6.

Schumacher, E.F. (1995) *A Guide for the Perplexed*, Vintage, London.

<table>
<tr><td>

5

</td><td>

Is homoeopathic prescribing reliable?

</td></tr>
</table>

Peter Fisher

INTRODUCTION

The year 1996 was the 200th anniversary of homoeopathy: the word 'homoöpathie' was coined by the Saxon physician Samuel Hahnemann in his essay 'on a new curative principle', originally published in *Hufeland's Journal* in 1796 (Hahnemann, 1851). In this seminal article, Hahnemann described three methods of healing. The first is removing or destroying the causes of the disease; this Hahnemann described as the 'Royal Road to healing', but as not always feasible. The second and most widely used is *contraria contrariis*, healing opposite by opposite. It was on this second method that Hahnemann focused his critique, writing, 'I ask my colleagues to desert this way: it is the wrong one, a false path in the gloomy forest which leads to the abyss.' He argued that in chronic diseases, or diseases that might become chronic, *contraria contrariis* might give short-term relief but in the long term made matters worse. His third method of healing is the diametric opposite of *contraria contrariis* – the treatment of like with like, *similia similibus curentur* – on the grounds that 'One should imitate nature, which, at times, heals a chronic disease by another additional one'.

This idea had been planted in Hahnemann's mind some years earlier while he was translating into German a materia medica written by the Edinburgh professor Cullen. China, or cinchona, the bark of the tree *Cinchona officinalis*, is the source of quinine, and was something of a miracle drug at the time. It is an effective treatment for malaria, which was then common in parts of Europe. Cullen claimed that it was effective because of its tonic effect on the stomach. Hahnemann criticised this view in his translator's notes, and went on to describe the symptoms he developed after he took 'four drams of good

China, twice a day'. He developed 'all those symptoms which to me are typical of intermittent fever, such as the stupefaction of the senses, . . . but above all the numb, disagreeable sensation which seems to have its seat in the periosteum of all the bones of the body' (Haehl, 1922).

The historical precedents of modern homoeopathy are extensive. The opposing ideas of using medicines on the basis either of similarity or of opposition were first explicitly raised, at least in the Western medical tradition, around 450 BC in the Hippocratic work 'On the places in Man' (Hippocrates, 1839–1861). Specific examples of similarity in the Hippocratic corpus include the use of the purgative Helleborus (*Veratrum album*) to treat cholera (Hippocrates, 1839–1861) and cantharis (*Cantharis vesicatoria* or 'Spanish fly'), which is highly toxic to the urinary tract, as a diuretic (Hippocrates, 1839–61).

The Hippocratic corpus also includes examples of an earlier non-physiological 'magical similarity', such as the use of the red juice of the pomegranate to treat bleeding. Magical similarity is a form of sympathetic magic, which is extremely widespread in primitive societies, carrying the idea of similarity or analogy back to the earliest human societies. In his classic work, *The Golden Bough* (1907), Sir James Frazer describes 'Charms based on the Law of Similarity (which) may be called Homoeopathic or Imitative Magic.'

Another important precursor of homoeopathy was the Swiss Renaissance doctor, alchemist and iconoclast Philippus Theophrastus Bombastus von Hohenheim (1493–1541), better known as Paracelsus. He advocated the doctrine of signatures, a form of primitive magical similarity, according to which every medicine, if studied closely enough, would yield a clue or 'signature' revealing its use. So, the bitter-tasting, yellow juice of the greater celandine (*Chelidonium majus*) resembles bile, indicating that the plant is a medicine for jaundice. The black, shiny berries of the deadly nightshade (*Atropa belladonna*) resemble the dilated pupils of patients with fevers that will respond to it.

Another strand in the historical antecedents of homoeopathy is represented by Mithridates the Great (King Mithridates VI Eupator, 132–63 BC), known as the 'Father of Toxicology' (toxicology is the science of poisons). At the end of his long struggle with the Romans, Mithridates found himself besieged and attempted to kill himself with poison. He took a massive dose, sufficient to kill several men, but it failed to kill him. Eventually he had to order one of his own soldiers to behead him. The secret of Mithridates' resistance to poison foreshadows homoeopathy: every day he took a special formula, consisting of small amounts of all known poisons, thus inducing what we would now call an adaptive response, making him highly resistant to poison. This formula, known as mithridatum, remained in use in Europe well into the nineteenth century (Watson, 1966).

EXPERIMENTATION: HAHNEMANN'S ADVANCE

If Hahnemann was not the originator of the idea of treatment on the basis of similarity, what was his original contribution? It was that he was the first to insist on pathophysiological similarity rather than magical similarity or the doctrine of signatures. Logically, if medicines are to be used on the basis of pathophysiological similarity, one must first know the pathophysiological effects they induce in healthy people. This led Hahnemann to develop the method known as 'proving' (the word is a translation of the German 'prüfung', meaning 'test'; 'homoeopathic pathogenetic trial' (HPT) has recently been proposed as a more accurate term) (Dantas, 1996). In a proving the substance of interest is given to healthy volunteers and their symptoms are recorded. Hahnemann gathered together a band of provers, many of them doctors interested in the new method and, with them, proved a wide range of substances. The first collection of 70 provings, of substances ranging from the highly toxic, such as arsenic, to the mundane *Taraxacum* (dandelion) was published in Hahnemann's *Materia Medica Pura* (1825–1830).

It is difficult for us now to appreciate just how revolutionary Hahnemann's methods were at the end of the eighteenth century. Although his conclusions had been foreshadowed in the views of others, it was the method by which he reached them that was remarkable. His use of medicines was based on experiment, rather than received wisdom. Throughout his life, Hahnemann remained sceptical of physiological and therapeutic theories. Instead he treated the body and its ills as a 'black box', whose input (medicines) and output (symptoms) were knowable but whose internal workings were unknown. Although he does not seem to have believed that the body's internal functioning is inherently unknowable, he insisted that 'the totality of symptoms and circumstances observed in each individual case is the one and only indication that can guide us to the choice of the remedy' (Hahnemann, 1982).

Hahnemann was harshly critical of his medical contemporaries, accusing them of killing, gradually, more millions than Napoleon ever slew in battle. Contemporary conventional doctors retaliated in turn, but on surprising grounds, accusing the early homoeopaths of empiricism, in other words of relying on experience rather than 'rational' principles. Ironically, in the intervening two centuries, the position has reversed, and it is now medical orthodoxy which aspires, to base its treatments on evidence, while homoeopathy all too often relies on information of dubious provenance and reliability, or outdated dogma.

THE VALIDITY OF PROVINGS

Although an historic advance, these early provings suffered from important weaknesses, which raise fundamental questions about their validity. The most important is that they were uncontrolled, meaning that there was no comparison group. Thus there is no way of knowing whether the symptoms recorded really related to the medicine being taken by the volunteers, or whether they resulted from more careful self-observation by the provers, or would have occurred anyway. These problems are illustrated by one of Hahnemann's own original band of provers, the neurotic and suggestible Langhammer (Bodman, 1987).

Later provings or HPTs have adopted some degree of placebo control, but this has generally been inadequate, typically involving a small proportion of the volunteers taking placebo (an indistinguishable preparation lacking the active ingredient), while the remainder take the active preparation. The problem with such a methodology is that there is no intra-individual control. Homoeopathic treatment is highly individualised: its success depends crucially on the sensitivity and idiosyncrasy of the individual patient. Suppose that, in a group of 20 volunteers, two were sensitive to the substance, and that one of them received placebo, the other active medication. The placebo volunteer might report symptoms, due to closer self-observation, expectation or inter-current illness. The volunteer in the active group would develop symptoms, but there would be no way of knowing whether these related to the medicine or were due to closer self-observation, expectation or intercurrent illness. The solution to this problem may be a crossover method, whereby all provers take both the active and placebo preparations in a double-blind, randomised fashion, so that if some volunteers consistently develop certain symptoms when taking the active but not the placebo medication, one can be sure that the volunteer is sensitive and the symptoms do relate to the medicine. This method does have problems, including 'order effects' (volunteers tend to report fewer symptoms as time goes on) and possible 'carry over effects' (effects from treatment might 'carry over' into the placebo period).

Homeopathic pathogenetic trials continue to be done. In recent times more have been done and published in the UK than anywhere else in the world: 45 in the 50 years from 1945 to 1995. A recent systematic review of HPTs has showed wide variation in methodology, for instance the number of volunteers ranged from 1 to 103 (Dantas and Fisher, 1998). But perhaps the most alarming finding was that the number of symptoms reported as associated with the medicine fell off sharply with improving quality of the HPT, so that the best HPTs, from the methodological point of view, reported few, if any, symptoms (Clover *et al.*, 1980; Walach, 1993).

HOMOEOPATHIC PRESCRIBING AND THE REPERTORY

The problem of the logical structure of homoeopathic prescribing decisions can be traced right back to Hahnemann, and his repeated insistence that homoeopathic medicines should be selected on the basis of the totality of symptoms. Very little consideration has been given to the logical structure of the processes leading to an individualised prescription based on a 'totality of symptoms'.

The basis of individualised prescribing decisions for many homoeopaths is the repertory. A repertory is simply a list of symptoms. Hahnemann developed his own small repertory, simply an *aide-mémoire* of symptoms. The first full scale repertory was published by Boenninghausen in 1832. Ironically, although various repertories were widely used by homoeopaths from this time on, because of the sheer amount of information processing involved, full potential of the method was not realised until the development of the personal computer 150 years later. Because of the number of medicines listed against each symptom, even a simple repertorisation such as that shown in Figure 5.1 would be far too time consuming to perform in a busy practice, while a large scale repertorisation such as that represented by Figure 5.2, involving 22 symptoms, would involve several hours work if done manually. Repertorisation thus lends itself to information technology, and computerised repertories and decision support systems started to emerge in the early 1980s, soon after the introduction of the personal computer. Punched card repertories had been developed in the 1960s, but they never achieved wide popularity.

The most enduring contribution to homoeopathy of the 'high' school (homoeopaths using high dilutions) has been Kent's Repertory (Kent, 1973)

	Belladonna	Aconite	Stramonium	Chamomilla
Mind Delirium	3	2	3	2
Ear Inflammation inside	3	2	–	3
Face Discolouration red	3	3	3	3
Generalities Sudden	3	3	3	–
Sum of degrees	12	10	9	8

Figure 5.1. Repertorisation of a case of acute otitis media, using the Synthesis repertory and Radar software. The numbers indicate how strongly a medicine is associated with a particular symptom (3 = strong association, 1 = weak). Some repertories use 4 'degrees' of association. In this analysis, mental and general symptoms have not been given extra weighting, but the software could be set to do this. Compare this with Figures 5.2 and 5.3. This repertorisation suggests that belladonna is the indicated medicine.

(a)

Medicines	A	B	C	D	Number of symptoms
Symptom Rank	2	3	4	1	2
	3	4	2	1	12
	4	1	2	3	8
Total	**72**	**62**	**48**	**38**	

(b)

Medicines	A	B	C	D
A	–	8	20	22
B	14	–	12	14
C	2	10	–	14
D	0	8	8	–

Figure 5.2. (a) The sum of degrees method applied to homoeopathic repertorisation: four medicines (A,B,C,D) are compared on 22 symptoms. They are ranked according to which is most strongly indicated for each symptom: A is elected/prescribed. (b) The pairwise majority method applied to homoeopathic repertorisation using the same data as (a): A scores more highly than B for 8 symptoms, B more highly than A for 14 symptoms and so on. The final result is B>A>C>D. B is elected/prescribed.

and its descendants. The evolution of the repertory is now largely electronic: the main computerised repertory programs currently used in the UK are CARA, MacRepertory and RADAR*. Each of these incorporates its own expanded version of Kent's Repertory and other databases. The Synthesis Repertory linked to the RADAR program and the Complete Repertory linked to MacRepertory both exist in printed form (Schroyens, 1995; Van Zandvoort, 1994–1996). These descendants of Kent's repertory are massive works: for instance, the latest edition of the Synthesis Repertory is a book of over 1800 pages, containing over 600,000 items of information, occupying some 12 Mb of disk space.

While the software is powerful and user friendly, the fundamental problem of information technology – 'Garbage in, garbage out' – has not been solved. As Campbell has shown, many symptoms listed in the repertory cannot be

*CARA for Windows (Miccant, Nottingham). MacRepertory for Macintosh and Windows, (Kent Homeopathic Associates, Fairfax, CA). Radar for Windows and Macintosh Archibel, (Assesse, Belgium).

traced to HPTs, particularly for 'constitutional' homoeopathic medicines, which are prescribed on the basis of particular types of personality and general features rather than syndromes. For instance, *Rhus toxicodendron* (poison ivy) is one of the most commonly used homoeopathic medicines, mostly for rheumatic and arthritic problems. It was originally proved by Hahnemann on ten volunteers, including himself; he also drew up on a number of other authors and included a total of 976 symptoms (Hahnemann, 1825–1830). A number of other nineteenth century provings of *Rhus toxicodendron* were compiled by Hughes (1891). As would be expected from its known effects, most of the symptoms were in the skin, although some musculoskeletal symptoms were reported. The drug picture on the basis of which it is now prescribed does emerge reasonably clearly from the provings (Campbell, 1981a). The same cannot be said for other commonly used homoeopathic medicines. For instance, the homoeopathic medicine lycopodium – derived from the spores of the club moss *Lycopodium clavatum*, and also proved by Hahnemann, with further documentation by Hughes has evolved an elaborate drug picture, with numerous mental and 'constitutional' features, but the provings generated relatively few, nondescript symptoms.

It is clear that most of the picture of this homoeopathic medicine has accrued through clinical experience (Bodman, 1936; Campbell, 1981b). But, in the case of Kent's Repertory, for most symptoms, we have no idea who observed which symptoms to be cured in which disease under what circumstances. This information appears to have been lost, if, indeed, it was ever recorded. Some of the modern repertories list the sources of all new information added, but most of the information is simply carried over from Kent, and there is no standardisation of criteria for the addition of new symptoms.

In short, the knowledge base of homoeopathy is seriously flawed: the methodology of HPTs has generally been poor, and likely to have resulted in an inflated number of symptoms attributed to medicines. Worse still, most symptoms used in practice do not derive from HPTs at all, but from clinical experience. Frequently we do not know the provenance of the clinical experience, and, where it is recorded, the criteria for attributing symptoms to the medicine are not standardised. Again, the net effect is to inflate the number of symptoms associated with medicines. Given these fundamental flaws in the knowledge on which homoeopathic prescribing is based, it is perhaps surprising that homoeopaths practise successfully and that the evidence from controlled clinical trials is positive. The reason may lie in the way in which real-life prescribing decisions are made in homoeopathy.

THE LOGIC OF HOMOEOPATHIC PRESCRIBING

In Kent's Repertory and its descendants, the first chapter is 'Mind', and the last is 'Generalities'; the intervening chapters are organised anatomically, with a few exceptions (e.g. 'Stool', which follows 'Rectum', or 'Fever'). Within each chapter, information is grouped into 'rubrics', which list the medicines associated with a particular symptom, and 'subrubrics', for instance subdividing pain according to its character. Medicines are listed by 'degree', indicating how strongly they are associated with a particular symptom. 'Synthesis' (a widely used modern repertory) uses four degrees, denoted by normal, italic, bold and capital type, where normal type indicates a weak association and capitals a very strong one (see Figure 5.1). (Note that degree is here used in a different sense from Swedenborg's doctrine of degrees.) There is no standardisation of qualification criteria for different degrees, although Synthesis has degree criteria for data from a few sources.

What of the 'totality of symptoms'? It is in the construction of 'totality of symptoms' that the unacknowledged Swedenborgian influence persists most strongly in contemporary homoeopathy, although most homoeopaths are unaware of it, and even shocked when it is pointed out. Yet the influence is plain, and seen most clearly in Kent's insistence on a hierarchy of symptoms: mental symptoms are of the greatest significance, followed by general symptoms and finally particular symptoms. Within the mental symptoms there is a subhierarchy, the most important being 'loves and hates', followed by symptoms relating to reason and then memory. This doctrine was reiterated by the influential British homoeopaths Dr Margaret Tyler and Sir John Weir, who were not Swedenborgians (Tyler, 1973). As van Galen has shown, this doctrine reflects Swedenborg's philosophy precisely (van Galen, 1994).

Given the weakness of the information in repertories, it is unlikely that prescribing based entirely on repertorisation would be very successful, and it is clear that homoeopaths do use other methods to make prescribing decisions. In recent years there have been some attempts to analyse the decision-making process in homoeopathic prescribing. Essentially, the homoeopath compares two sets of data: the symptom set which he collects by talking to the patient, and the symptom sets of different homoeopathic medicines, as recorded in the repertory. As Fichefet has pointed out, this process is analogous to an election: the medicine that scores the maximum number of matches between its symptoms, as listed in the repertory and those of the patient wins the election, and is prescribed. But it is not quite as simple as that: in repertories, homoeopathic medicines are listed in 'degrees', indicating how strongly they are associated with a particular symptom; and there are several systems of election.

Systems of election include: simple majority; ranking or Borda's method, in which each elector ranks the candidates in order of preference; and pairwise majority or Condorcet's method, in which the electors state a preference between every pair of candidates. The application of different methods to repertorisation can lead to different decisions (see Figure 5.2). Mathematical theory predicts that a skilled homoeopath is more likely to find the right medicine using the pairwise majority method than is a less skilled one (Fichefet, 1992).

Algorithms provide a pragmatic alternative to repertorisation for decision support in homoeopathic prescribing, and a number of such algorithms have been developed. Van Haselen and Liagre have developed decision trees for homoeopathic prescribing in otitis media (see Figure 5.3), which illustrate some important points. Symptoms may be context specific, so that the prescribing indication 'irritable' can lead to different prescriptions in different contexts, while the prescribing decision 'Pulsatilla' can be reached by two different routes. Algorithms provide a useful model of homoeopathic prescribing but can only be sustained within very limited domains, as indicated by the dead 'other medicine' branches of the decision tree (van Haselen and Liagre, 1992).

Although the two methods described above – repertorial election and decision algorithm provide adequate descriptions of certain types of homoeopathic prescribing decisions, both suffer from serious weaknesses and it is clear that neither is a comprehensive description of the logical structure of the prescribing decisions made by experienced homoeopaths. Apart from the deficiencies in the data, and the hidden ideological assumptions of the Repertory, the method is not truly holistic. The whole is more than the sum of its parts, but the repertorial method is just that: a summation of symptoms. Similarly a single channel algorithm is not holistic.

On a more practical level, both methods are very vulnerable to distortion by a single symptom. For instance, what is 'sudden onset' (Figures 5.1 and 5.3)? Does it mean onset in seconds, minutes or hours? A more frequent problem is translating the symptoms as related by the patient, or features observed by the prescriber, into repertory rubrics. For instance, the rubric 'Ear: pain in children' might quite legitimately be included (provided, of course, the patient was a child), or used instead of 'Ear: inflammation' (especially at an early stage in the illness, before the inflammation was evident) in the repertorisation shown in Figure 5.1. But although the rubric 'Ear: pain in children' includes the second and fourth remedies suggested, Aconite and Chamomilla, it does not contain the first choice, Belladonna. In this way, slightly different repertorial interpretations of the same symptoms might lead to quite different prescriptions.

In fact most homoeopathic prescribing is not done on the basis of formal repertorisation. Most experienced British homoeopaths use a repertory sparingly, rarely performing a full repertorisation, using it instead to check a few symptoms. Indeed, before the advent of personal computers it would have been impractical to use it in any other way. Yet practical homoeopathic prescribing is much more robust, and less likely to be blown of course by the interpretation of a single symptom than would be suggested by the problems discussed above.

How is this achieved? The answer appears to be that the process by which an experienced homoeopath reaches his or her prescribing decisions is more holistic than the assumptions of these models. The homoeopath looks for an overall

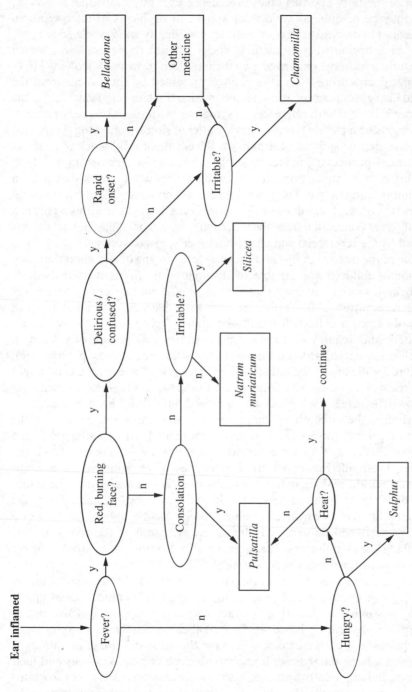

Figure 5.3. Part of a flowchart for homoeopathic prescribing in acute otitis media. Adapted from van Haselen and Liagre (1992). Key: ◯ = decision node; y = yes; n = no; ▢ = prescribing decision.

pattern or 'gestalt', and this takes precedence over any individual symptom, which may be of dubious validity or subject to problems of interpretation. Experienced homoeopaths report that they confidently anticipate a good result from a prescription when 'something clicks' – when they recognise a match between the syndrome picture of a medicine – derived from toxicology, HPTs and clinical experience – and the picture, presented by the patient from the medical history and examination. Homoeopaths think in very visual terms, the literature is littered with references to symptom pictures and remedy pictures, and recognising a picture is more than a matter of simply compiling symptoms; it involves the recognition of a pattern. Recent theoretical work in artificial intelligence – particularly in inductive, classifier and visual recognition systems – has interesting implications in this context. This work shows that pattern recognition requires 'parallel processing', in which information from several sources is processed simultaneously before being brought together. This is a quite different conception from the simple summation or single channel models assumed by the repertorial and algorithm models, respectively.

Some of the interest in this area was triggered by the observation that even very young children are capable of distinguishing different animals quite reliably and, more important, that they have efficient learning processes for animal recognition. After only one encounter with an animal it has not previously seen, a child will usually be able to recognise the same species accurately and reliably in future. Furthermore, children quickly learn to generalise: animals of widely differing shapes, sizes and colours can all be dogs.

Figure 5.4 illustrates the inductive logic processes that a young child might use to recognise and classify animals. At this stage, there is not enough data to know whether a small black creature without a long head is a cat or a squirrel. But the strength of characteristics may carry the child over the decision threshold (a very small animal is more likely to be a squirrel than a cat), (see Figure 5.4(b)). Or a further stage may be required to reach the decision threshold (Figure 5.4(c)). This process of recognition can be compared to decision making in homoeopathy: the visual cues become the symptoms, their strength the degrees, and the different types of animals are the medicines. Similarly hearing an animal – which was thought to be a cat or a squirrel – bark is like a so-called 'eliminative symptom' in the homoeopathic prescribing decision process. The presence of an 'eliminative symptom' forces the decision process to go back one stage (Figure 5.4.(c)).

Such inductive models are a fascinating future line for the understanding of the logic of homoeopathic prescribing decisions. This model opens up the exciting possibility of providing interactive decision support systems for homoeopathic prescribing based on large, validated databases of symptoms, prescriptions and their outcomes. Perhaps the most intriguing possibility is that, given a large database of homoeopathic prescribing decisions and their outcomes, inductive software could learn which decision paths were associated with positive outcomes. The incorporation of a so-called 'bucket brigade'

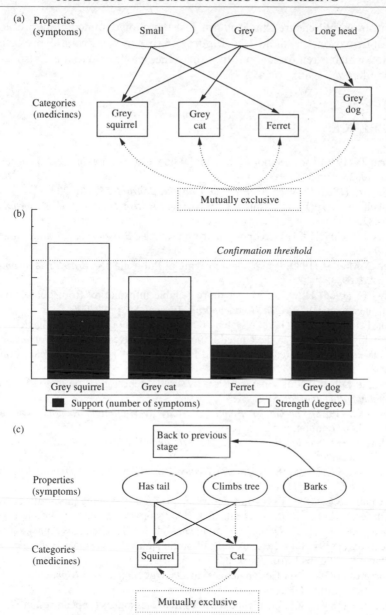

Figure 5.4. (a) Inductive recognition model for animals. (b) Although the categorical data is insufficient to decide whether a small grey creature with a short head is a cat or squirrel, the strength of the properties may allow confirmation: a very small animal is more likely to be a squirrel. (c) Alternatively, more categorical data can be gathered. Again, a cat may climb trees, but a squirrel is more likely. However, if a small animal with a rounded head barks, it may be a Pekinese dog! If such an 'eliminative feature' is observed, the process goes back one stage. In terms of homoeopathic prescribing decisions, properties are analogous to symptoms, their strength to degrees and categories to medicines.

algorithm would ensure that it is not just the choice immediately preceding the confirmation threshold (see Figure 5.4.(b)) of a successful prescribing decision which is reinforced, but that the stages leading up to it are also learnt (Holland *et al.*, 1986).

REFERENCES

Bodman, F. (1936) The evolution of the Lycopodium drug picture. *British Homoeopathic Journal*, **26**, 416–33.
Bodman, F. (1964) Provers. *British Homoeopathic Journal*, **53**, 161–70.
Campbell, A.C.H. (1981a) Rhus from provings. *British Homoeopathic Journal*, **70**, 179–82.
Campbell, A.C.H. (1981b) Lycopodium from provings. *British Homoeopathic Journal*, **70**, 94–9.
Clover, A.M *et al.* (1980) Report on a proving of Pulsatilla 3X. *British Homoeopathic Journal*, **69**, 134–49.
Dantas, F. (1966) How can we get more reliable information from homoeopathic pathogenetic trials? *British Homoeopathic Journal*, **85**, pp. 230–6
Dantas, F. and Fisher, P. (1998) A systematic review of homoeopathic pathogenetic trials ('provings') published in the United Kingdom from 1945 to 1995, in *Homoeopathy: an objective proposal*, (eds E. Ernst and E. Hahn), Butterworth Heineman, London (1998).
Fichefet, J. (1992) About some traps set by 'crude' repertorization methods. *British Homoeopathic Journal*, **81**, 2–12.
Frazer, J.G. (1907) *The Golden Bough: A Study in Magic and Religion*, volume 1, Macmillan, London, p. 52.
Haehl, R. (1922) *Samuel Hahnemann: His Life and Work*, Homoeopathic Publishing Co., London.
Hahnemann, S.C. (1825–1830) *Materia Medica Pura* (trans. R.E. Dudgeon). Reprinted by Jain & Co. New Delhi.
Hahnemann, S.C. (1851) Essay on a new principle for ascertaining the curative powers of drugs, in *Lesser Writings*, (trans. R.E. Dudgeon), W. Headland, London.
Hahnemann, S.C. (1982) *Organon of Medicine*, 6th edn Tarcher, Los Angeles.
Hippocrates (1839–1861) Des lieux dans l'homme, in *Oeuvres complètes d'Hippocrate*, volume 6, Editions Littré, Paris, pp. 334–5.
Hippocrates (1839–1861) Des epidémies, in *Oeuvres complètes d'Hippocrate*, volume 5, Editions Littré, Paris, pp. 210–11.
Hippocrates (1839–1861) De régime dans les maladies aigues (appendice), in *Oeuvres complètes d'Hippocrate*, volume 2, Editions Littré, Paris pp. 512–13.
Holland, J.H. Holyoak, K.J. Nisbett, R.E. and Thagard, P.R. *Induction*, MIT Press, Cambridge MA.
Hughes, R. (1891) *Cyclopaedia of Drug Pathogenesy*, volume 4, E. Gould and Son, London.
Kent, J.T. (1973) *Repertory of Homoeopathic Materia Medica*, Hahnemann Publishing, Calcutta.
Schroyens, F. (1995) *Synthesis 5.2 ed.*, Homoeopathic Book Publishers, London.

Tyler, M. (1973) A study of Kent's Repertory, in Kent, J.T. *Repertory of Homoeopathic Materia Medica*, Hahnemann Publishing, Calcutta.

van Galen, E. (1994) Kent's hidden links. *Homoeopathic Links*, **7**, 27–38.

van Haselen, R.A. and Liagre, R. (1992) Systematic investigation of the decision process in homoeopathy. *British Homoeopathic Journal*, **81**, 13–17.

van Zandvoort, R. (1994–1996) *The Complete Repertory*, Institute for Research in Homoeopathy, Leidschendam.

Walach, H. (1993) Does a homoeopathic drug act as a placebo? *Journal of Pychosomatic Research*, **37**, 851–60.

Watson, G. (1966) *Theriac and Mithridatum*, Wellcome, London.

| 6 | **Complementary therapies: complementing nursing?** |

Caroline Stevensen

INTRODUCTION

There appears to be increasing interest in complementary therapies among nurses in the UK. This is not unproblematic. In this chapter, complementary medicine within nursing will be examined in the light of the various assumptions, claims and behaviours of nurses about the use of these therapies in their profession. For example, it may be assumed that nurses who use complementary therapies are more caring and that their approach to nursing is more holistic. Nurses also refer to the 'energetic' benefits of complementary medicine, without understanding. Explanations given by nurses for the mechanisms and effects of complementary treatments given may border on the magical or esoteric, which risks alienating nurses who practise complementary therapies from the rest of the profession who seek a base of rational evidence for clinical practice. There are questions about which therapies are appropriate for which patients and – a danger that nurses may offer one complementary therapy to all patients because that is the only available therapy in a given clinical area.

The overall intention of this chapter is to help nurses to challenge some underlying assumptions about the practice of complementary medicine in nursing.

THE RANGE OF COMPLEMENTARY THERAPIES WITHIN NURSING

Let us begin with the question of which aspects of complementary medicine nurses are actually practising. The term 'complementary medicine' is often used in nursing as if nurses were using a range of therapies. In fact, surveys examining the use of complementary therapies amongst nurses (Rankin Box and Stevensen, 1997; Trevelyan, 1996) show that nurses mainly use a narrow band of complementary therapies. These include primarily massage, aromatherapy and reflexology. Less often nurses use other therapies including Therapeutic Touch, relaxation and visualisation techniques, shiatsu, acupuncture, hypnotherapy, homoeopathy and herbalism.

This has some interesting corollaries. Nurses need to examine decisions about the provision of complementary medicine. As the majority of nurses are training in massage, aromatherapy and reflexology, this must mean that patients are primarily offered these therapies. This limited range of therapies is cause for concern. It is quite possible that none of these therapies is the therapy of choice for a wide range of patients in any given clinical situation and that may mean that these patients are offered no complementary therapies or only those less appropriate ones that are available. In choosing which complementary therapies to practise, nurses need to question their motivation, the needs of the patients in their clinical setting, and which therapies may be most appropriate for these patients, and then offer as broad a range of therapy options as is practical.

The questions of how these complementary therapies fit into the professional nursing role and what nurses consider to be acceptable also need to be addressed. Nursing has often been referred to as the caring profession, with images of Florence Nightingale and her lamp, of nurses mopping fevered brows with undivided attention and holding the hands of dying patients. There is, however, no evidence to show that nurses are more caring than other professionals or indeed that the kind of care and attention offered by nurses would be better offered in another way. The addition of complementary therapies, including those therapies using touch has been seen by nurses as a natural extension of their caring role, however, little evidence currently exists on how far complementary therapies might enhance that role. The use of both technical and caring touch has traditionally been part of nursing practice and many of the therapies chosen by nurses involve touch of some kind.

THE USE OF TOUCH THERAPIES BY NURSES

In general, touch in nursing has been viewed as an acceptable means of offering comfort and support to patients and carers. The balance between the administration of technical and caring touch in nursing practice has been a key topic of discussion in recent years, with the development of an increasingly technological approach to many branches of nursing. It is assumed that there should be, where possible, a balance between the technical and caring aspects of touch in nursing care, although the thinking behind this is based on the idea that patients who are in highly technological medical environments such as intensive care are generally deprived of caring and therapeutic forms of touch. In practice this may well be the case.

It may be difficult for nurses to achieve this balance between caring and technical touch due to the pressure on professional time to meet the demands imposed by the highly technological environments in which they work. This problem has led many nurses to wish to use hands-on therapies to attempt to redress this balance. Sound evidence for the benefit of these touch therapies presently remains under-researched. The 'feel good factor' and relief of symptoms in patients receiving complementary therapies are what most nurses rely up on as evidence of worthwhile practice. The number of quality clinical trials in massage, aromatherapy and reflexology performed by nurses in the UK is very few, and the evidence from these is not necessarily conclusive (Corner, Cawley and Hildebrand, 1995; Dale and Cornwell, 1994; Dunn, Sleep and Collett, 1995; Stevensen, 1994; Wilkinson, 1995). This still then leaves questionable assumptions about the level of benefit of these hands-on therapies to patients. Common sense tells us that there are likely to be some positive effects for patients, but lack of comparative analysis about methods of delivery using touch therapies may leave some doubt as to how much benefit is actually derived.

HEALING POTENTIAL OF COMPLEMENTARY THERAPIES

In searching for the rationale for the healing effectiveness of complementary therapy practices, some nurses are turning to explanations from the traditional philosophies of India and China. These philosophies give explanations for the practice of acupuncture, shiatsu, reflexology and Reiki from the Chinese tradition and yoga relaxation, breathing and visualisation exercises, based in the Indian tradition. In these philosophies there is claimed to be a life force or vital energy, known as *chi* in traditional Chinese medicine or *prana* in Indian philosophy. Nurses claim to influence these vital body energies during their practices of complementary therapies.

It may be difficult for nurses to rationalise their practice according to such theories in a professional environment steeped in Western medical science. Moreover, what is meant by healing may vary. From a scientific viewpoint, success in the 'balancing of the patient's energies' may be difficult for a nurse to discuss with colleagues.

Unless the healing response or reaction is clearly defined, it is difficult for nurses to ascertain exactly what changes they are achieving using complementary therapies. What may be healing for one patient may not be considered healing for another. Nurses need to be careful with their use of terminology and in making claims about the results of any complementary treatments.

ENERGETIC EFFECTS OF COMPLEMENTARY THERAPIES

Nurses using complementary therapies often use the term 'energy', referring to its modulation and enhancement via the practice of complementary therapies. The difficulty is that there is no clear concept of exactly what this energy is. 'Energy' as described by complementary therapists is not necessarily tangible. The 'rebalancing of the body's energy fields' is referred to in the practice of Therapeutic Touch, while 'rebalancing the meridian energy' – using acupuncture, shiatsu or reflexology – or 'balancing the chakras' – using breathing or visualisation – are explanations taken from the ancient systems of healing such as yoga and traditional Chinese medicine, to explain the effects of the complementary therapies.

One consideration is that nurses, who have traditionally had less scientific training than their medical colleagues, may be more open to esoteric ideas about the use of subtle body energies, for which scientific evidence is difficult to secure. It has happened in recent years that some nurses using esoteric explanations for their practice of complementary therapies have been prevented from using them by their professional colleagues, who regard them as unscientific.

POTENTIAL BENEFITS OF COMPLEMENTARY THERAPIES

Claims about the potential benefits of complementary therapies need to be viewed with caution due to the absence of a substantial clinical research base. Therapies such as acupuncture and homoeopathy are less shaky in their evidence base, by virtue of the number of quality clinical trials conducted on them. There are several hundred clinical trials on acupuncture and homoeopathy (Royal London Homoeopathic Hospital, 1997), compared to less than ten in aromatherapy, about four in reflexology, and a wealth of rather poorly conducted trials in massage which do not enable a fair analysis of its benefits (Vickers, 1996). This lack of a proven scientific rationale for complementary therapies does not assist nurses with implementing them in the orthodox clinical setting.

Even the therapies most commonly adopted by nurses, including aromatherapy and reflexology, cannot offer a sure explanation for their mechanisms of action on a scientific basis. Many nurses wishing to practise complementary therapies in their clinical environments go to managers with as much research as they can find and with evidence of their use in other clinical environments, only to be told that these complementary therapies are unacceptable, unproven or potentially unsafe. Lack of available research into essential oils is one example where a number of hospitals have banned the practice of aromatherapy, fearing adverse interactions or side effects from the treatments. Managers and purchasers of health care have power over the implementation of complementary therapies. As with any change or development in nursing, there may be opposition to the introduction of new therapies which is based on the lack of research evidence or their unacceptability to professional colleagues. Fortunately, as more and more patients are recounting positive and helpful experiences from complementary therapies, such views are necessarily being examined. It may be argued, given the current lack of a large body of research evidence for these therapies, that managers are justified in their decisions not to allow the practice of these therapies in clinical areas. It could also be argued that it is the responsibility of each individual nurse practising a complementary therapy to audit and research the work that they are doing in order to increase the available body of evidence.

COMPLEMENTARY THERAPIES IN NURSING: WHO BENEFITS?

It is always important to examine the motivation for any professional practice, and the use of complementary therapies in nursing is no exception. For the patient, complementary therapies may provide symptomatic relief, an overall sense of well-being and quality of life support that have not previously been offered via conventional means.

However, the use of complementary therapies in nursing may also lead us to address certain problems with which nurses and nursing practice are struggling. It is fair to ask who gains more benefit from the therapies – the nurses or the patients? The use of complementary therapies may be rekindling some aspects of nursing where the ability to truly care for the patient has been thought lost. Complementary therapies may offer a positive identification with and expression of the nursing role. From this angle, it may also be suggested that nurses learn and practise complementary therapies for their own personal and professional growth and their own self healing, not merely from an altruistic perspective on patient care.

On the negative side, is it possible that complementary therapies will be viewed as just another task, being performed by nurses already overstretched in their duties with the automatic precision of some of the more technical or fundamental tasks in nursing?

Should there be concern that using complementary therapies in clinical practice seems to offer so much for the nurse or should this be welcomed as a positive step forward for the profession? If nurses are gaining so much from delivering the therapies, does this enhance the quality of the care received by patients? Are complementary therapies as valuable to the patient as to the nurse providing it? All these questions warrant further examination. As the nurse grows and develops and gains more satisfaction in her role, it is hoped that the quality of patient care also improves, but there is currently little evidence to confirm that this is necessarily the case for the practice of complementary therapies.

LENGTH AND TIMING OF COMPLEMENTARY THERAPY TREATMENTS

The length and timing of treatments practised by nurses is another controversial area in complementary medicine. The optimal interval of time between treatments is also debated among therapists. How do nurses ascertain the optimal treatment regime for any patients receiving complementary therapies? At present there appears to be no research examining the length of treatments in any of the major complementary therapies practised by nurses. Rather than being limited by set appointment times and lengths, nurses may choose to vary the length of treatments according to individual need. Not many nurses practice complementary therapies full time in their job, so these therapies may need to be fitted around a number of other responsibilities and tasks. Advocates of certain therapies recommend certain set times for their practice. In some forms of meditation, such as Transcendental Meditation (TM), the recommended pattern of practice is 20 minutes, 2–3 times per day. Autogenic Training, a systematic method of relaxation, also recommends three sessions per day. Advocates of other relaxation/meditation techniques claim that, once a technique has been learnt, only three minutes three times per day will allow the individual to reach a profound state of relaxation. How then can nurse therapists make decisions as to the optimal length of time for their patients? In the absence of formal research, nurses must make decisions according to their own assessment of individual patients in conjunction with the patient themselves.

For the hands-on therapies, there is no evidence to suggest that one hour of massage is necessarily better for the individual than, say, 20 minutes. It may also be that the use of appropriate local techniques over a shorter length of time, such as massage for the relief of stiff and painful shoulders, may have generalised effects in the body as a whole and at a psychological level. Again, nurses must assess each patient as an individual to obtain the information required to assess the optimal length of time and appropriate kind of treatment.

In practice, reflexology is often recommended twice per week, massage, aromatherapy and shiatsu once per week, and relaxation anything from several times per day to weekly. There may also be a danger of overloading the patient with too lengthy or too frequent treatments, not allowing the body's innate healing mechanisms to take effect. Here again the decisions rest in the hands of the therapist. In the case of debilitated and fatigued patients, excessive treatment may lead to worsening of the patient's overall condition. There is currently no overall agreement in any field of complementary medicine about the length and frequency of treatments. The individual variation of both practitioners and patients no doubt plays some part in this. It is rare in the current economic climate that the nurse can offer an optimal number of complementary treatments, due to increased clinical demands and time constraints and limited funding. This forces the question of whether nurses should be providing a service that is less than optimal, where the maximum benefits to patients may not be reached.

DOSAGE AND ROUTE OF ADMINISTRATION OF SUBSTANCES

Another difficulty that nurses face is knowing what may be regarded as the correct dosage and route of administration of substances used in complementary medicine. In the absence of an agreed formulary for the prescribing of essential oils, homoeopathic medicines or herbal substances, optimal dosages have not been confirmed. The homoeopathic literature does not agree on what is the exact dosages for any prescriptions, nor does the literature pertaining to aromatherapy and the use of essential oils. Individual practitioners administer these medicines according to accepted practice, but much of this practice is inconsistent and does not have a research basis.

Essential oils may be inhaled, massaged into the skin, applied in a compress, placed in a bath or taken internally. Some aromatherapists claim that essential oils have properties that blend synergistically with each other when mixed, thus creating a more powerful effect than one oil alone. Other aromatherapists claim that the higher the level of essential oil in the prescription (within safe limits), the more powerful the clinical effect. Many claims made in the currently available range of aromatherapy textbooks are unsubstantiated. Nurses are in a difficult position to know exactly what is safe and what is an optimal dosage and route of administration for essential oils. Dosage of essential oils varies from book to book, with no research results absolutely confirmed in any text for many of the oils commonly used in aromatherapy. Nurses using these essential oils have little idea whether the dose used is correct for the individual patient, a situation that would not be tolerated in conventional pharmacology. Until the natural substances used in complementary medicine are investigated, the answers to these questions will not be known. Due to the enormous cost of doing such research, it is unlikely that comprehensive data will be available in the foreseeable future.

This may leave nurses at risk of either not recommending to patients the correct doses of homoeopathic medicines or essential oils to gain optimum therapeutic value or, conversely, of putting the patient at risk due to excessive administration. Nurses would be wise to err on the side of caution, but in the process may not administer enough of the substances for them to be clinically effective.

CONTRAINDICATIONS TO COMPLEMENTARY THERAPIES

The issue of contraindications to complementary therapies is another dilemma faced by nurses practising these therapies. Common sense may tell practitioners not to massage over broken limbs, or to try relaxation techniques on a patient who is in a psychotic state, or to stimulate certain points of the body. The exact dangers of essential oils are not well researched and the use of many oils is based on assumptions about their properties and their effects on the body. The side effects or dangers of essential oils mentioned in the literature are based on the use of large doses of essential oils usually tested in animal or tissue models, with few human clinical trials. Until well conducted clinical trials are performed for each oil, safety and therapeutic data will remain inadequate. For other therapies such as reflexology, assumptions about practices are based on empirical evidence of their effects and side effects, with little really known, in the absence of research about the impact of the therapy on the body as a whole. Teachers and practitioners of these therapies are in danger of generalising the side effects of these therapies from the experience of an individual patient, which could lead to drawing false conclusions. Nurses need to be clear and logical in their discussion with patients about these important matters in order for the patients to gain benefit from hands-on therapies.

HOLISTIC PRACTICE?

The word 'holistic' is one used by many nurses practising complementary therapies but its exact meaning is not always clear. It has been said to refer to an approach towards patients which addresses physical, mental, emotional and spiritual needs. This is often contrasted with conventional medicine, which is said to take a reductionist and segmented approach to health, where individual problems are regarded with little reference to the patient as a whole.

But, though many nurses who practise complementary therapies claim to operate from a holistic perspective, this may or may not really be true in clinical practice. For example, complementary therapies are sometimes used by nurses to relieve local symptoms, such as the use of massage or acupressure to relieve a headache. In what sense are complementary therapies more holistic than say, aspirin, in such a context?

It is also necessary to question how the benefits of holism are measured. Does having a holistic approach enhance the care that is being given, or is it purely in the minds of the nurses practising complementary therapies that this is the case? The effects of complementary therapy treatments may not be seen immediately after a session has finished and the impact on that person's life – positive or negative – may never be known in holistic terms by the nurse. The same may be true in other areas of professional nursing practice, which, increasingly, is aiming to be holistic in its approach. The concept of a therapeutic relationship with patients is only beginning to be explored by nurses. We have yet to see the full impact this may have on the range of interactions between patients and nurses including the practice of complementary therapies.

CONCLUSION

In embracing complementary therapies as part of their professional nursing practice, the nurse is faced with many questions and dilemmas. While patients' demands for complementary therapies are increasing, so are the number of nurses training in and practising a narrow band of therapies. Nurses need to question the range of therapies they are practising and the ways that these may be of benefit to patients. The terminology used in complementary therapies needs to be viewed with caution. 'Energy' and 'holism' are examples of words that are used more often than they are understood. Explanation of the mechanisms by which the therapies work is another area where nurses should tread with caution. Nurses need to question assumptions about the benefits of complementary therapies and look at their motivation for practising these therapies. Another challenge is to find out from a sound evidence base the optimal administration times, frequencies and doses and contraindications related to complementary therapies. In their desire to provide quality complementary therapies, nurses need to ask themselves whether they are using the therapies purely as techniques – or whether a more holistic approach has been adopted. Whatever the outcome to all these questions, nurses using complementary therapies need to practise with a greater degree of critical self-appraisal.

REFERENCES

Corner, J., Cawley, N. and Hildebrand, S. (1995) An evaluation of the use of massage and essential oils on the wellbeing of cancer patients. *International Journal of Palliative Nursing*, 1(2), 67–73.

Dale, A. and Cornwell, S. (1994) The role of lavender oil in relieving perineal discomfort following childbirth: a blind, randomised clinical trial. *Journal of Advanced Nursing*, 19, 89–96.

Dunn, C. Sleep, J. and Collett, D. (1995) Sensing an improvement: an experimental study to evaluate the use of aromatherapy, massage and periods of rest in an intensive care unit. *Journal of Advanced Nursing*, 21(1), 34–40.

Rankin Box, D. (1997) Therapies in practice: a survey assessing nurses' use of complementary therapies. *Complementary Therapies in Nursing and Midwifery*, 3, 92–9.

Royal London Homoeopathic Hospital (1997) Evidence base of complementary therapies. Royal London Homoeopathic Hospital NHS Trust, London.

Stevensen, C. (1994) The psychophysiological effects of aromatherapy massage following cardiac surgery. *Complementary Therapies in Medicine*, **2**(1), 27–35.

Trevelyan, J. 1996 A true complement? *Nursing Times*, **92**, 42–3.

Wilkinson, S. (1995) Aromatherapy and massage in palliative care. *International Journal of Palliative Nursing*, **1**(1), 21–30.

Vickers, A. (1996) *Massage and aromatherapy: a guide for health professionals.* Chapman & Hall, London.

7	# Principles or practice? An exploration of the role of theory in homoeopathy

Bob Fordham

For merely looking at an object cannot be of any use to us. All looking goes over into an observing, all observing into a reflecting, all reflecting into a connecting, and so one can say with every attentive look we cast into the world we are already theorising.

Goethe (Walsh, 1993)

The suffering of the morbidly mistuned, spirit-like dynamis (life force) enlivening our body in the invisible interior, and the complex of the outwardly perceptible symptoms portraying the present malady, which are organized by the dynamis in the organism, form a whole. They are one and the same. The organism is indeed a material instrument for life, but it is not conceivable without the life imparted to it by the instinctual, feeling and regulating dynamis, just as the life force is not conceivable without the organism. Consequently, the two of them constitute a unity, although in thought, we split this unity into two concepts in order to conceptualize it more easily.

Hahnemann (1842)

INTRODUCTION

To assert general truths is to impose a spurious dogma on the chaos of phenomena.

Tarnas (1991)

This chapter is an exploration of the general truths of homoeopathy and of the variety of homeopathic phenomena. More specifically, it is an exploration of the uneasy – and largely unexplored – tension between the two.

Homeopaths relate the success of homoeopathy as a medical system to its adherence to natural laws and to its respect for the natural healing effort of the organism. Accordingly, I explore the homeopathic view of natural laws and vitalism as a key central principle of homeopathic philosophy. I am interested in how our central ideas influence the way we practise and the potential distorting effects of homeopathic principles. Two key questions are addressed. First, does our knowledge of the principles of homoeopathy exert a distorting influence on practice? Second, do we idealise the phenomena of practice to fit our principles?

Principles and laws are stable. Practice and, indeed progress, imply change and flexibility. Homeopaths have acknowledged this tension in different ways. The first – Hahnemann's approach – was to derive set of universal laws or principles which would encompass and explain clinical phenomena. He relied on the elegance of the system he devised to demonstrate its validity. The second approach has been to appeal to the authority of science and scientific approaches. This has, to my mind, created an unsatisfactory scientism within homoeopathy.

Homeopathic philosophy consists of those ideas that homeopaths hold to be true and which enrich, sustain and inform practice. In much the same way that teachers articulate an educational philosophy, anyone engaged in a practical discipline will embody, and act upon, their personal version of a broader philosophy which encompasses what is generally held to be true within their discipline. Practice involves managing a series of unique events, each patient and each prescription being seen as individual. It should not be surprising that it is difficult to subsume these phenomena under broad principles.

While my concern in this chapter is homoeopathy, I believe the discussion presented here will interest all who are concerned to advance a debate on the place of theory in the practice of complementary medicine. This has personal relevance to me as a practitioner. I well remember the impact homeopathic principles had on me. I was immediately impressed by a challenging view of health, disease and medicine. Homeopathic ideas resonated with my understanding as a biologist, enabling me to grasp the central significance of symptoms as a potentially homeostatic mechanism. The appeal lay in the elegance, simplicity and coherence of its philosophy. It answered many of my own questions clearly and convincingly. I was also impressed because the philosophical poverty of allopathic medicine was exposed – I had been struggling with that for some time. However, the longer I practise and teach homoeopathy, the more I find my initial assessment of homeopathic principles somewhat cosy and uncritical. This essay is an attempt to relocate my initial acceptance of homoeopathy within a critical debate.

UNIVERSAL PRINCIPLES AND THE AUTHORITY OF HOMEOPATHIC KNOWLEDGE

Homeopathic philosophy carefully and accurately defines a general approach to health and disease. Homeopaths are – justifiably, in my view – proud of the robustness of their philosophy. Coulter (1982, p. 475) states:

> the homeopathic doctrine is stable and has never suffered the upheavals observed in the history of Rationalist medicine . . . these physicians have not been led astray by will-o-the-wisps of vaunted discoveries which . . . are seen to be much less beneficial than was at first assumed.

In any discipline, some statements are more authoritative than others. All systems of thought need to establish the basis of authority, to describe how it is possible to make significant contributions to knowledge. The authority of homoeopathy has generally been seen to rest on the capacity of its principles to organise and explain the phenomena of health, disease and cure. Hahnemann said, 'The highest ideal of cure is the rapid, gentle and permanent restoration of health . . . according to *clearly realisable principles*.' (1842, p. 60; emphasis added.)

The centrality of therapeutic principles in homoeopathy is difficult to overstate. Harris Coulter (1980, p. 18) summarises:

> Homoeopathy differs from allopathy in possessing a precise set of principles governing diagnosis and treatment. The physician who does not follow these principles more or less accurately cannot be said to practice homoeopathy . . . homoeopathy has always adhered to a set of assumptions about the functioning of the human organism in health and disease, the nature of its relationship to the external world, and the effects of the medicines used to treat disease. Since these assumptions are quite precise, the rules of homeopathic practice are also precise.

Vithoulkas says it is necessary to ask, 'What are the laws and principles governing the function of the human being in health and disease?' (1980, p. 13.) This view is axiomatic in homoeopathy. Writing in the preface of his repertory, Jansen (1992, p. i) makes a typical statement:

> We should never forget that obstetrics, pregnancy, childbirth and the puerperal period are natural processes. Attempting to control these subtle biological events could interfere with the fundamental laws of nature, possibly complicating the situation and making even more stringent control necessary.

As homeopaths, we state that our principles represent valid insights into the fundamental behaviour of living organisms in health and disease. These insights imply that natural laws govern these processes. Homeopathic practice should respect them and work in harmony with them.

I have said that homeopathic principles express a view of health and disease which is both highly coherent and cogent. Their coherence – the power they have to synthesise many ideas into stable propositions – contributes to their cogency. That poses a problem. It may become an invitation to suspend criticism and judgement, to interpret the clinical observations according to principle, rather than critically appraise a spectrum of possibilities. Furthermore, the process of interpretation, the activity of the practitioner in observing and evaluating clinical information, is barely acknowledged.

A SCIENTIFIC MEDICINE?

If a claim to universal principles offers one way of approaching the validity of homeopathic knowledge, an appeal to science offers another. Coulter (1982, p. 488) gives this explanation of its basis:

> Support for the scientific status of homoeopathy is found in the realisation that its knowledge is stable and cumulative . . . Carol Dunham in 1885 defined a scientific medicine as one possessing the 'capability of infinite progress in each of its elements without detriment to its integrity as a whole.'

When I first encountered homoeopathy I would have heartily agreed with a statement of Blackie's used to preface an edited collection of her writing and teaching – in *Classical Homoeopathy* (1986):

> Homoeopathy, as formulated by Hahnemann, is the most scientific and the most successful system of medical treatment yet devised. Our responsibility for its pure and truthful presentation is great.

Now, having taught homoeopathy to student-practitioners for about eight years, life does not seem so simple.

While Dunham's view of a scientific medicine might have been appropriate to the late nineteenth century, would it pass the test of late twentieth century scientific orthodoxy? On what grounds is homoeopathy 'the most scientific' system of medical treatment? On what grounds is it scientific at all? Can orthodox scientific measures be successfully applied to classical homeopathic practice? Is it the 'most successful system' of medical treatment? How do we know? Is it possible to present it 'purely and truthfully'? Should I, in my role as a teacher, attempt to present Hahnemann's ideas? Can I separate them from my own experience as a practitioner? Clearly, an appeal to science raises more questions than it answers.

How do we avoid polarising a dogmatic insistence on principle with a *laissez-faire* approach to practice and the introduction of new ideas?

When we approach homoeopathy as a dynamic and evolving system of medicine, such questions become urgent. I am interested in why homeopaths have adopted this 'scientific' characterisation of homoeopathy and the impact this has on discussion of the subject. This debate has recently received a stimulus from George Vithoulkas (1995, p. 4), who has launched a vehement attack on the 'artistic distortions' which he sees as arising in the imagination of some homeopaths:

> We have had a lot of problems persuading people that homoeopathy is a *Science*. Now, with all this nonsense, we are once again reinforcing their arguments claiming that Homeopathy is a 'non-science'. Such ideas . . . are signs of *degeneration* in our science, *the results of which we will soon be witnessing.*' (Emphasis in the original.)

For me this statement bypasses issues of real importance. It presents science and scientific enquiry as essentially unproblematic. Science is accorded special status and acquires the role of arbiter. That is, scientific validity is validity *per se*, which seems to me at best, optimistic or epistemologically naïve, at worst simply untrue. A searching enquiry into the validity of homeopathic ideas needs to account for interpretation, for the practitioner's imagination and aesthetic sense. It cannot simply seek to proscribe such issues by defining the rules for the discussion in narrowly scientific terms.

Some attempts to characterise artistic perception seem to me to be highly appropriate to complementary practice. For example, Shklovsky (quoted in Aston and Savona, 1991, p. 7) said, 'Art exists that one may recover the sensation of life; it exists to make one feel things, to make the stone *stony*.' The qualities of the stone have thus become more accessible to the observer, not distorted. As practitioners, are we not equally striving to achieve a similarly insightful characterisation of illness?

Therapies differ in their particular approaches, language and concepts, but all are united in seeking to present a coherent basis for practice, to articulate a general philosophy that guides practitioners. We work with individuals. The philosophy seeks to generalise clinical experience, to articulate what is usually true and reliable. When the philosophy 'works' it applies to the particular case in question. The therapeutic intervention – derived from those broad principles – also 'works' and the patient improves. The practitioner predicts a beneficial outcome and that is what follows. The philosophy is thereby validated. Note, however that this is not a scientific process, in the narrow sense of 'scientific' as defined by, say Karl Popper, who argued that science progressed not by seeking verification but by constructing theories which are gradually adapted to more robust forms under a sustained and rigorous attempt to refute them.

Homeopathic philosophy offers a stable and challenging general perspective on health and disease. It serves to define the imperatives of practice in general terms and provides a reference point from which practitioners consider practical problems. While homeopaths have been clear about what is stable in their philosophy – the principles – they are less certain about how to reconcile 'infinite progress in each of its elements' with these unchanging ground rules. I think Dunham's statement is entirely appropriate to the needs of homoeopathy, allowing as it does for the refinement of homeopathic knowledge.

It is now time to address the creative tension that arises between these different aspects of homeopathic knowledge.

PRINCIPLES IN PRACTICE

Previously I described a situation in which the overall philosophy proved a successful guide to practice. A second outcome for the broad philosophy exists. It may fail the practitioner, and thereby the patient. Practitioners re-evaluate their approach at this point. Is this a crisis? No. The demands of practice require that the general philosophical approach is refined and adapted to essentially unique circumstances. Every patient and every consultation is different. This requires creativity. I would guess the delight that most of us experience as practitioners comes not from our ability to enact skills from well rehearsed routines, but from our engagement with the unique qualities of each individual clinical problem and in applying our knowledge flexibly. Note again that, while that process may be characterised in robust and rigorous terms – it is not orthodox science. Rigorous descriptions of professional knowledge and its application do exist (see Eraut; 1994 Schön, 1983, 1987). Homeopaths and others will find useful insights in these texts to help characterise practitioner knowledge.

For me, the growth and development of our philosophy come from the testing and adaptation of general concepts to unique clinical situations. In this way our knowledge is refined. Scientific procedures are not well suited to a sustained exploration of this kind of process. I hope we can redefine our search for a rigorous approach to studying homoeopathy. For such an enquiry to be meaningful we need to adopt methods that yield reliable and valid information in the homeopathic context. It is an error to graft scientific methodology – developed to answer questions in a different field of human endeavour – on to our own. Unless we wish to limit the kinds of questions it is permissible to ask, we must adopt methods relevant to our own needs, to the kinds of questions homeopaths seek to answer and to the unique knowledge base of homoeopathy.

Let us stop for a moment to consider how these principles arise. The raw data of homoeopathy are vast, comprising information on poisonings, provings and published case histories. Practitioners will add to this the personal knowledge and insights gained through their own clinical experience. It is impossible to approach this volume of information without some organising mechanism. The principles serve to organise these observations into a coherent whole. They provide a consistent means to consider homeopathic problems. One cannot stop and consider the plethora of individual observations. The practitioner must synthesise these into their own working philosophy. Clinical observation and evaluation represent the acting out of this personal philosophy in relation to the case under consideration. Practitioners will draw on many faculties in order to evaluate cases. They are looking for form, pattern and meaning. It is not unusual for practitioners to use adjectives that relate to the aesthetic qualities they perceive as the jumble of symptoms in a case history begins to take shape.

However, homeopaths make a further claim for their principles. Their consistency suggests they represent valid statements about the laws of nature. These statements have a powerful rhetorical effect and are much more problematic, in my view. First, I am uncertain how we can know that this is the case, though we may choose to believe it to be true. Second, this notion can – in my opinion – constrain how practitioners view cases. It invites them to impose a form or pattern on the material of the case history, which is then interpreted as evidence of an underlying process obeying a natural law: if we suggest a natural law, then surely the organism is going to obey it? At this point the power of the overarching philosophy to organise a *general* view of health and disease can exert a distorting influence by creating unrealistic expectations of each individual situation. The activity of any single case may not be referable to general principles. To attempt to do so is to favour a particular interpretation of the patient's history on *a priori* grounds.

I began this piece with the quote from Goethe because it stresses the importance of the observer in organising observations into theories. He stresses the subjective experience of the observer. Goethe also said 'the phenomenon is the theory', implying it is unnecessary to theorise beyond the observations themselves. His is a science of the subjective. The appeal to natural law is a positivist position. It implies that there is a real organising force which may be described or revealed and that this accounts for the phenomena observed. Note that the observer and the processes of observation and evaluation of the material observed, are missing from this view. From this perspective, natural laws govern the phenomena we perceive. They proceed from a substantial, objective basis. It seems to me that homoeopathy has failed to grasp the tension between these two points of view. Homeopaths have consistently sought to validate their data – which are arrived at subjectively – by reference to a positivist framework: the existence of an organising factor.

THE IMPLICATIONS FOR HOMOEOPATHY

I would like to illustrate the consequences of this, using the homeopathic concept of the vital force, or *dynamis*, as an example.

The quote from Hahnemann at the head of this chapter describes a reductionist process at work. In order to comprehend the activity of the organism we invent mental categories. The organism, which he understood as a unity, is divided into a 'material instrument for life' and its *dynamis* in the attempt to describe the phenomena. He clearly identifies the *dynamis* as an artefact. It is created in the act of comprehending. This has been a perennial problem for Western thinking, expressing as it does an analogous duality to that between mind and body.

In his monograph *Homeopathic Medicine*, Coulter (1972, p. 4), emphasises the centrality of vitalism for homoeopathy:

> From Hahnemann onwards, the homeopathic physicians have charac-terised the processes of health and disease in vitalistic terms . . . This reactive power is manifested in the symptoms of disease, just as it also makes its presence felt in the rhythmic alterations of the body's functions in health . . . the vitalistic assumption is of primordial importance for homeopathic therapeutics, since it imposes a particular interpretation of the symptom . . . [as] the visible manifestation of the organism's reactive power.

This observation influences the practitioner's view of therapeutics. To quote Coulter again, 'The curative medicine is the one which supports and stimulates the organism's incipient and inchoate healing effort.' (Coulter, 1972, p. 4.)

These statements involve a rewriting of homeopathic history. The symp-toms are the primary data. Hahnemann did not formally incorporate a vitalist view into his work until he wrote the fifth edition of the *Organon* (1842). His early writings display an impatience with the idea: 'At one time, men created for themselves an imaginary incorporeal something, which guided and ruled the whole system in the vicissitudes of health and disease,' he wrote in 1808 (Hahnemann, 1851).

What Hahnemann observed was that a remedy that produces symptoms X, Y and Z will cure an illness that has the symptoms X, Y and Z. This observation alone has tremendous implications for the practice of medicine. The role of the remedy is to mimic the illness, eliciting a reaction in the organism. The enhanced reaction of the organism overcomes the illness. Is the existence of the vital force central to this perception? I would say not; after all, physiologists describe essentially similar processes in the homeostatic behaviour of living things without the need to refer to a vital force.

Why has homoeopathy adopted vitalist doctrine? Hahnemann expresses one reason. In discussing the behaviour of the organism it is a matter of ease of comprehension, but he acknowledges that this is a shorthand, a conven-ience. But there is probably another process at work. When we perceive patterns in phenomena, we assume there is a substantial, objective basis for those patterns, that is, a pattern maker. We anticipate a natural force behaving according to natural law and we find one. Furthermore we deny the relevance of the subjective experience and the conscious creative effort of both patient and practitioner in constructing knowledge when we do so. Kent (1900) reinforced this view for a new generation of homeopaths, and Vithoulkas

(1980) continues the tradition. He has named this organising power the defence mechanism but its position in homeopathic philosophy is unchallenged.

I reiterate the concern that the uncritical acceptance of this can lead us – in the clinic – to prefer answers that appear to obey 'the rules' to those that are not so obvious. We may distort our observations to fit preconceived notions of what is acceptable according to perceived natural law.

I have experienced this myself as a tutor of homoeopathy. We taught our students a series of models with which to evaluate case histories. We illustrated these with case examples. The model and the case were well matched. Students were given exercises to do which reinforced the models. Some time later our students began to ask us, 'Why do you teach us these ideas when we do not see you use them yourselves in teaching clinics?' This came as quite a surprise. What we had done is created a set of idealised patterns. These 'work' when the appropriate, archetypal cases come along, but what of the rest? We were forced to consider how we applied this information ourselves. In fact, we seem to apply the models flexibly. We add elements of one model to another and combine other homeopathic information until we have created a story, an image, a pattern that is meaningful in a holistic sense. Set against the background of the continuous variability we see human experience and suffering, our models represent arbitrary categories. They are more helpful when acknowledged as such.

IDEALISATION AND THE REAL WORLD OF HOMOEOPATHIC PRACTICE

We find the same process at work in other areas of homoeopathy. Sankaran (1991, p. 80) describes the relationship between homeopathic potency and symptoms in highly idealised terms:

> In low potencies *Nit ac* produces anxiety in the prover. This is unassociated anxiety, free floating anxiety with some irritability. When we go to the 30th potency, the anxiety becomes a little more specific . . . as we go higher to the 50,000th potency, the delusion is that he is fighting a court battle, that he is engaged in a long standing war in which he cannot yield comes to him quite clearly. So, one can say, as the potency increases the delusion becomes clearer and the original situation of the state is more clearly revealed.

My search of the proving material fails to find a basis for this statement, though I recognise the homeopathic orthodoxy expressed. In describing the application of potency in his materia medica of *Natrum mur*, Kent (1904) said, 'We may need to go higher and higher until the secret spring is touched.' This idealised view is usefully contrasted with observations made in a recent proving (Sherr and Preston, no date):

. . . of interest was the observation that detectable physical symptoms often appeared before detectable mental symptoms, therefore dispelling the idea that mental and emotional symptoms always appear first.

Francis Treuherz (1983) describes James Tyler Kent (1849–1916) as 'the ultimate homoeopath of the period when homoeopathy flourished in America'. His influence can be noted in the work of many modern homeopaths. Kent was a follower of the teachings of the Christian mystic Emanuel Swedenborg (see Treuherz, 1983). Kent's religious ideas influenced his writing about homoeopathy, though probably less so his practice. For me, his philosophy represents an idealisation of his homoeopathic work, in which he is motivated to recast homeopathic philosophy according to a Swedenborgian religious view. His case work (published posthumously in *Lesser Writings* (1951)) seems more influenced by Hahnemann. Kent felt the need to express a coherent philosophy influenced by Swedenborg's ideas. This is not clearly discernible in the published cases. Kent (1900, p. 68) records Hahnemann's adoption of a vitalist explanation in this way: 'Hahnemann could perceive this immaterial vital principle. It was something he arrived at himself, from his own process of thinking.' Contrast this with Wood (1992), who succinctly locates Hahnemann's change in his practice: 'Hahnemann became more amenable to the idea of vitalism. It explained homeopathic phenomena better.' Flexibility was anathema to Kent, who propounded rigid adherence to fixed laws. Not so for Hahnemann, who appears to have been more comfortable with notions of change and development of his doctrine.

Hahnemann observed, in paragraph 7 of the first edition of *Organon* 1810: 'There must be a healing principle present in medicines . . .' By 1893, when the fifth edition was published, he had clearly identified the healing principle with the organism. This represents the adaptation of principle to practice. Hahnemann was able to say both 'the truth of the homoeopathic healing art . . . can no longer be obscured . . .'; and: 'I have not refrained from making any alterations . . . necessitated by further experience.' (Hahnemann, 1893).

Barney Glaser (1978, p. 4) says

Being doctrinaire, and revering 'great men' interferes both with sensitivity to the data and with generating those ideas that fit and work best. It interferes because the assumption is one of forming the data to fit the doctrine.

I believe it will become increasingly important for homeopaths to account for the manner in which practice challenges principle. This will be facilitated by an appreciation that the models or maps we make to help us explore the patient's experience are constructed by the practitioner ('the map is not the territory'). Practitioners will hopefully begin to acknowledge and articulate their own role as map makers as they explore an unfolding clinical picture.

Our failure to do so has deprived us of a potentially rich and insightful discourse on the relationship between theory and practice in homoeopathy. Exciting and relevant possibilities exist. To paraphrase Davis, Sumara and Kieren, (1996), practice expresses a dynamic interplay of practitioner and patient which refuses to separate knowledge and activity and involves both mind and body. Practice and self-identity cannot therefore be separated. The exploration of homeopaths' doing, knowing and being should clearly expose the rhetoric of practice and open the way for a richer, clearer and more unified understanding of homeopathic knowing.

CONCLUSIONS

Homeopathic philosophy has been remarkably consistent. Hahnemann's principles are still the cornerstones of classical homeopathic philosophy. As a general explanation of health and disease they represent a powerful challenge to allopathic ideas. However, they tend to create an expectation of idealised patterns in the behaviour of the human organism in health and disease, particularly when coupled to the concept of an organism manifesting behaviour or symptoms according to an underlying natural law. Anticipation of such idealised behaviour in practitioners can influence their clinical perception.

If classical homoeopathy is to be studied critically it will require careful attention to the application of homeopathic knowledge in practice. The way that homeopaths and their patients collaborate in constructing a meaningful image of the illness is likely to be a fruitful area for study. It will be important to describe how homeopaths apply their analytical tools and models. I personally believe that homeopaths themselves must carry out this work. If this happens we can anticipate the emergence of a robust description and analysis of our professional knowledge. This should mitigate against any gap between theory – the homoeopathy of books and journals – and practice as we experience it daily in the clinic. We may then find that the coherence of homeopathic principles at a general level can be extended to incorporate the fine details of practice.

REFERENCES

Aston, E. and Savona, G. (1991) *Theatre as sign system*, Routledge, London.
Blackie, M. (1986) *Classical Homœopathy*, (eds C. Elliot and F. Johnson), Beaconsfield Publishers Ltd., UK.
Coulter, H. (1972) *Homœopathic Medicine*, Formur & American Foundation for Homœopathy, St. Louis.
Coulter, H. (1980) *Homœopathic Science and Modern Medicine*, North Atlantic Books, Berkeley, CA.

Coulter, H. (1982) *Divided Legacy – The Conflict between Homœopathy and the American Medical Association*, North Atlantic Books, Richmond, CA.

Davis, A.B., Sumara, D.J. and Kieren, T.E. (1996) Cognition, co-emergence, curriculum. *Journal of Curriculum Studies*, **28**(2), 151–69.

Eraut, M. (1994) Professional knowledge: its character, development and use, in *Developing Professional Knowledge and Competence*, Falmer, Lewes.

Glaser, B. (1978) *Theoretical Sensitivity*, Sociology Press, Mill Valley, CA.

Hahnemann, S. (1808) On the value of the speculative systems of medicine, in *Hahnemann's Lesser Writings*. (Trans. R.E. Dudgeon), Jain, New Delhi.

Hahnemann, S. (1842) *Organon of Medicine*, 6th edn. (Trans. S. Decker; ed. W.B. O'Reilly, 1996), Birdcage Books, Redmond.

Hahnemann, S. (1893) *The Organon of Medicine*, 5th edn. (Trans. R.E. Dudgeon). Reprinted, 1985, Jain, New Delhi.

Jansen, J.W. (1992) *Synthetic Bedside Repertory for Gestation, Childbirth and Childbed*, Merlijn, Haarlem.

Kent, J.T. (1900) *Lectures on Homœopathic Philosophy*, Reprinted 1982, Jain, New Delhi.

Kent, J.T. (1904) *Lectures on Homœopathic Materia Medica*, Reprinted 1982, Jain, New Delhi.

Sankaran, R. (1991) *The Spirit of Homoeopathy*, Sankaran, Bombay.

Schön, D.A. (1983) *The Reflective Practitioner*, Basic Books, New York.

Schön, D.A. (1987) *Educating the Reflective Practitioner*, Jossey-Bass, San Francisco.

Sherr, J. and Preston, R. (no date) *The Homeopathic Proving of Hydrogen*. Dynamis School, West Malvern.

Tarnas, R. (1991) *The Passion of the Western Mind*, Pimlico, London.

Treuherz, F. (1983) Hecla Lava (or the influence of Swedenborg on Homœopathy). *The Homœopath*, **4**(2), 35–53.

Vithoulkas, G. (1980) *The Science of Homœopathy*, Grove Press, New York.

Vithoulkas, G. (1995) Homeopathy: art or science? *European Journal of Classical Homeopathy*, **1**(1), 3–5.

Walsh, P. (1993) *Education and Meaning*, Cassell, London, p. 71.

Wood, M. (1992) *The Magical Staff: The Vitalist Tradition in Western Medicine*, North Atlantic Books, Berkeley, CA.

PART THREE

Beliefs

This section explores issues which are common to more than one form of complementary medicine. Clive Wood examines the concept of 'body energy' and argues that complementary practitioners may have mistaken the map for the territory. Just as we avoid saying that, for example, a content individual is full of 'contentment fluid', so we should avoid saying that a energetic individual has harmonious 'body energy'. The 'vital force' may best be thought of as metaphor rather than something which has a place in the physical world. Stephen Tyreman explores the relationship between conventional and complementary medicine using the specific example of osteopathy. He argues that practitioners have not consistently or coherently identified points of similarity and difference between osteopathy and biomedicine. This may be because osteopaths have been unable to define exactly what it is they do. Still's three principles are fairly meaningless when examined carefully and more recent definitions of osteopathy are so vague that they could be used to describe just about any field of medical practice. David Peters attacks the idea that complementary therapies are inherently holistic by pointing out that the concepts of 'complementary medicine' and 'holism' cannot be examined in isolation from wider social changes. There have been cultural shifts away from the belief that there is a single, predominantly scientific, way of describing the world and that technological advance is the hallmark of progress. Peters argues that many 'myths' about complementary medicine stem from a reaction against biomedicine following these cultural changes. Anthony Campbell offers a critique of commonly held assumptions about complementary therapies, including the idea that they are natural, traditional, anti-authoritarian, non-materialistic, and deal with causes rather than just symptoms. His main point is that though each of these assumptions is questionable, each meets a powerful psychological need.

<table>
<tr><td>

Subtle energy and the vital force in complementary medicine

</td><td>

8

</td></tr>
</table>

Clive Wood

> Conventional medicine is the only medical system which has ever existed that does not have a vitalistic approach to illness and does not contain any concept of biological energy. All other systems of medicine, including the so-called complementary or natural therapies have some concept of vital force or energy of some description.
>
> Kenyon (1994, p. 21)

INTRODUCTION

In that opening quote, Julian Kenyon succinctly expresses a fundamental belief that underlies the theory (if perhaps not always the practice) of many forms of complementary therapy. It is the notion that physiological and psychological states are dependent upon the existence of some underlying form of 'subtle' energy. It is an energy of a kind quite different from that recognised by conventional medicine. Balance at this subtle level produces a state of health. Imbalance in subtle energy is a precursor (even an actual cause) of subsequent disease. The role of the complementary therapist is to prevent such imbalance from occurring. If it has occurred, the therapeutic task is to correct or realign it, as a result of which the client's physical or mental state should also return towards normality.

The importance of such subtle energetics to complementary medicine can perhaps be judged from a feature article (Schreeve, 1988) in the *Journal of Alternative and Complementary Medicine* which declares that 'subtle energy – or the invisible "life force" – is as much taken for granted as a fundamental fact of healing . . . by alternative therapists as it is dismissed outright . . . by the orthodox scientific medical world.' The belief in a life force, the feature suggests, 'is fundamental to most natural therapies and this, they claim, links them directly to the mystery healing schools of the Middle and Far East, predating the Graeco-Roman Christian tradition from which modern medicine largely springs' (Schreeve, 1988, p. 17).

The purpose of this chapter is to explore the concept of 'vital force' as it is described in a number of complementary traditions. We consider some attempts that have been made to produce more 'objective' (i.e. instrumentally demonstrable) evidence of its existence and hence to create a rationale that would bring such an energetic concept within the framework of conventional science. Finally, we consider an alternative formulation in which the life force is conceptualised as an essentially subjective experience on the part of the client, but nonetheless one with considerable therapeutic potential. I suggest that the consistent failure to demonstrate a more objective basis to vitalism has and will continue to have surprisingly little effect on the everyday practice of those complementary therapies that invoke it.

THE CONCEPT OF THE LIFE FORCE IN SOME ALTERNATIVE THERAPIES

Kenyon (1994) is perhaps a little too dismissive of 'conventional medicine' in claiming that it has no concept of biological energy. I have suggested elsewhere (Wood, 1989, pp. 63–4) that all human life depends on solar energy trapped by plant chloroplasts during photosynthesis and utilised in the biochemical form of molecules like adenosine triphosphate. However, 'subtle energy' is apparently not to be confused with this more gross biochemical form. Nor is the term to be used in the psychoanalytic sense of the capacity to activate drives or motives (for example, to seek pleasure and avoid pain – see Pines, 1990). Instead of these notions of electron transfer or libidinal energy, the subtle energy (manifest for example in such forms as *qi* in Chinese or *prana* in Hindu medicine) has both a more universal and a more immanent quality.

For example, according to Seem and Kaplan (1987, p. 38) '*Qi* is matter on the verge of becoming energy, or energy at the point of materialising.' Similarly, the pranic energy of the Ayurvedic *doshas* occupies 'a place sandwiched between mind and body, where thought turns into matter' (Chopra, 1991, p. 25). Though *qi* and *prana* form the energetic substratum of the human body, both are more universal and all-pervading forces. Thus, for Leskowitz (1992, p. 64) 'All living beings are animated by and infused with a universal energy or consciousness . . . consciousness precedes matter and is not merely a by-product of material complexity, as is assumed in neurobiology.' And *prana*, whilst being the 'vital energy or life force that keeps the body alive and healthy', itself comes from three distinct sources: the sun, the air and the ground (Sui,

1990, p. 3–4). On entering the physical body these universal energies are channelled or concentrated in specific regions of the 'subtle anatomy'. Whilst *qi* flows in a complex set of channels or 'meridians', *prana* is concentrated in a series of seven rotating wheel-like or funnel-shaped *chakras*.

However, the energy field is not localised to the physical body. In pranic healing the energy body interpenetrates the visible physical body and extends beyond it some 4–5 inches. This invisible physical energy field which follows the contours of the visible body is called the *inner aura* (Sui, 1990, p. 9).

Many healers adopt a similar auric model. 'The Human Energy Field is the manifestation of universal energy that it is intimately involved with human life. It can be described as a luminous body that surrounds and interpenetrates the physical body, emits its own characteristic radiation and is usually called the "aura". . . . researchers have created theoretical models that divide the aura into several layers. These layers are sometimes called *bodies*, and they interpenetrate and surround each other in successive layers. Each succeeding body is composed of finer substances and higher "vibrations" than the body that it surrounds and interpenetrates' (Brennan, 1987, p. 41.) The healer's role is to work with these auric energies and, when they are disturbed, bring them back into balance and harmony.

Many other complementary therapies rely for their rationale on similar energetic or vitalistic concepts. In some, the connection is perhaps obvious. Thus, radionics, dowsing and crystal therapy all overtly depend on being able to access and utilise subtle energy sources not detectable by existing physical instruments. Perhaps less obvious is the vitalistic element in some other complementary therapies. For example, it is claimed that 'Homoeopathy has its basis in vitalism' (Leary, 1990, p. 114). Indeed, 'A hundred years ago vitalism saved homoeopathy, because it seemed to be the only thing that distinguished homoeopathic practices from the conventional medicine of the times' (Leary, 1990, p. 115). But Leary is opposed to the continued invoking of a 'vague vital force' as the rationale for homoeopathic practice. 'Because we cannot explain the action of a potency by known chemical or physical laws we do not have to produce a vital force for which we do not have one iota of evidence' (Leary, 1990, p. 116).

Aromatherapists have also drawn attention to the particular energetic value of 'natural' substances. Thus, 'over-refined food . . . is sadly lacking in life force' and, by contrast, natural, organic or untreated foods 'work in harmony with the forces within us' (Tisserand, 1977, p. 52). Alternatively, 'plants are living beings, each possessing its own energy potential which, according to the laws of nature, may be transmitted to us' (Ryman, 1984, p. 37).

Manipulative therapies may also claim that they achieve an intervention at the subtle level which accompanies or underlies their more gross physical procedures. Thus, acupressure and to some extent shiatsu base their practice on freeing the energy trapped or wrongly distributed within the body. Kinesiology also makes use of the concept of *qi* (LaTourelle, 1992). A significant number, perhaps the majority, of therapies classed as alternative or complementary therefore take some account of (and claim to influence) a more subtle energy level which surrounds and interpenetrates the human body. They include in their therapeutic practice some attempt to re-establish balance or harmony to an energetic (and hence to a physical) system that has become disturbed by a variety of pathogenic factors. These may be either internally generated (stress reactions, fear, alienation) or may impinge from outside (micro-organisms, toxins, pollutants).

These simple accounts of the nature of *qi* or *prana* do, of course, represent a gross simplification of far more complex philosophical systems. For example, traditional Chinese medicine (TCM) considers the polarity of the patient's energetic qualities (weak/strong, hot/cold, etc.) in terms of the *yin-yang* balance and the possible origin of the patient's disturbance in terms of five phases or elements (fire, earth, metal, water or wood). Only then does it consider the movement of energy in the twelve major and eight secondary energy channels or meridians (Seem and Kaplan, 1987, p. 20). But such complexity can lead to conceptual confusion. Having explored its historical origins, D.Z. Wu (1990) of the Shanghai College of TCM has described the notion of *qi* as 'badly defined and actually a compilation of three different philosophical concepts', which must make its therapeutic value somewhat dubious.

The notion of *prana* is also embedded in a complex philosophical system. Some would see the pranic system as representing a 'higher-order' model which encompasses much of the basis of TCM. According to David Tansley (1986, p. 6). 'The chakra system governs the meridians and acupuncture points. If there is an imbalance in a chakra, it will reflect into the acupuncture system and finally into the physical form.' According to Leskowitz (1992, p. 64) the *chakras* function as 'step down transformers [which] transduce universal life energy into physiologically usable chemical messages through the mediation of appropriate endocrine hormones'.

Clearly fundamental to this discussion of the function of the subtle life energy is the question of what exactly this energy consists of. Here we find total confusion. Stanley Jacobs (1989) has pointed to the difficulty in using the single word 'energy' to describe concepts as diverse as, on the one hand, the definition used by physicists (energy as the capacity to do work) and, on the other, an entity that springs 'from our own immortal unchanging self, that centre of pure consciousness, knowledge and bliss. Such spiritual energy is free, abundant and everywhere the same' (Jacobs 1989, pp. 97–8). So where does vital energy lic on this continuum?

CONCEPTUALISATION OF SUBTLE ENERGY IN COMPLEMENTARY MEDICINE

Therapeutic systems that invoke a 'vital force' – and according to Kenyon (1994 p. 21) this includes all currently practised systems other than Western medicine – appear to employ the practical, hands-on application of some all-pervading source of cosmic energy. This universal vital force can be transduced into and through the human body with health-promoting results.

The major conceptual problem here revolves around defining the nature of this universal energy. None of these alternative philosophical systems describes its nature in explicit, instrumentally testable terms. Indeed, is the subtle energy inherently detectable, or detectable only through its interactions with matter (in this case living tissue)? If the latter, then we can know little or nothing of its actual nature. In philosophical terms, such a position is perfectly tenable (like the Christian concept of 'supernatural grace'). But that position automatically precludes the design of any empirical, falsifiable experiments to explore its nature further. In so doing, it disqualifies itself from the world of instrumental investigation. In short, a subtle energy whose nature cannot be understood has more in common with a religious belief than a physical principle. This distinction is in no sense pejorative (either to religion or to physics) but it does seem inescapable.

Some alternative therapists have, however, suggested that subtle energy is a theoretically detectable physical entity, although our current detection systems are too crude to measure it.

Most of these attempts to characterise the life energy therefore relate it to some electromagnetic perspective, to produce a so-called 'bioelectronic' interpretation. For Glazewski (1989, p. 24) the living organism acts as an oscillator emitting a 'biological field of electromagnetic nature'. Such oscillations produce changes in charge density on the surface and 'This outer electron shell is an important agent in the organization of internal processors.' An alternative formulation has been to see the subtle energy as a somewhat more 'rarefied', but still instrumentally detectable field of 'bioplasma'.

The identification of vital energy as bioplasma has wide currency in some complementary medicine circles, although its definition is rarely clear. Thus, Sui (1990) declares that the term 'plasma' relates to 'the fourth state of matter . . . Plasma is ionised gas or gas with positive and negative charged particles . . . Science, with the use of Kirlian photography has rediscovered the bioplasmic body' (Sui, 1990, p. 6).

A more rigorous statement of this hypothesis is that 'the bioplasma associated with an organism comprises a matrix of elementary charged particles (e.g. free electrons and protons) which interpenetrates the gross molecular architecture of the organism and which maintains the morphological characteristics of the organism to the extent that when a minor section of the organism is excised, the bioplasmic matrix remains' (Quickenden and Tilbury, 1986, p. 90). If such a phenomenon existed in living organisms then they would show regions of semiconducting behaviour capable of changing the energy field in the immediately surrounding atmosphere. It has been suggested that this semiconducting activity may occur particularly in the cytoplasm and mitochondria.

The notion of the bioplasma has great appeal because it brings together ancient ideas of healing and modern quantum physics – currently a very popular mixture for alternative therapies seeking orthodox acceptance. But the theoretical basis for such a bioplasma is completely inadequate. Quickenden and Tilbury (1986) point out that (among other problems) such plasma conditions occur only in materials of high purity at low temperatures. The conditions in living cytoplasm are very different. While it is true that very weak patterns of electromagnetic activity can be detected beyond the human body, these are thought to result from changing patterns of physiological activity, for example in the heart, brain and nervous system. Rather than evidence for bioplasma, they simply represent 'the sum of the static and changing electrical and magnetic fields which surround a living organism as a result of these sorts of bodily activity'. The various hypotheses brought forward to justify the existence of the bioplasma 'are largely explicable in conventional terms' (Quickenden and Tilbury, 1986, p. 97).

EVIDENCE FOR THE EXISTENCE OF THE SUBTLE BODY

Since it does not conform to the established physical laws that describe electricity and magnetism, the vital force is some sort of 'non-conventional' electromagnetic phenomenon (perhaps with some quantum effects included). Not surprisingly, its demonstration and measurement are no easy task. Nonetheless, several lines of evidence are cited by complementary medicine practitioners in support of the demonstrable existence of a subtle energy body which is intimately associated with, but distinct from, the physical body and its more 'gross' and readily explained electromagnetic fields.

One of the most widely discussed is the use of Kirlian photography. On exposing living tissue (often a human hand) to a high-voltage, low-current field and capturing the effect on a photographic film, a complex discharge pattern or 'halo' can often be seen to surround the object on the photograph. While the outer part of the halo consisting of spiky protrusions is often quite spectacular, specialists in Kirlian methods are more interested in the inner portion which mirrors the shape of the object itself. A continuous inner image with few breaks in it is said to represent a more healthy subject than a discontinuous pattern with many breaks.

Many different discharge patterns are recognised and each allegedly has diagnostic value, being associated with some pathology that may be apparent in the Kirlian photograph before becoming diagnosable by any more conventional means. One suggestion is that the Kirlian image actually reflects the state of the bioplasma, and hence the individual's state of health. A more conventional explanation is that the high voltage field ionises molecules in the discharge path and that the resulting pattern has more to do with the subject's level of sympathetic arousal (and hence sweat-gland activity and skin resistance) than overall health status (Wood, 1986). No data correlating Kirlian diagnosis with other more conventional diagnostic methods seem to have been published and I am aware of no comparative trials of its value for diagnostic or therapeutic purposes.

Nor is the most widely quoted evidence linking the Kirlian image to the existence of a bioplasma particularly convincing. In the famous 'phantom leaf' experiment, a fresh leaf with a portion cut out of it is said to show a complete leaf-shaped Kirlian image because, although part of the physical structure has been removed, the bioplasmic 'aura' still remains. However, it is not so widely stated that such an effect is rarely reproducible, being obtained only once in hundreds or even thousands of trials (Quickenden and Tilbury, 1986, p. 99).

A second body of evidence allegedly pointing to the existence of subtle energy results from studies of acupuncture meridians, in which changes in electrical conductivity are traced along the surface of the body in pathways that correspond to the classical TCM meridian pattern, but not to any nervous pathways. The question of the existence and nature of acupuncture meridians is a large one, which is beyond our scope here. In a previous review I have suggested (Wood, 1993a) that, although the evidence for the efficacy of acupuncture in a limited number of therapeutic areas – and particularly in inducing analgesia – is well established, the existence of definable meridians, let alone the movement of subtle energy within them, is not. Even some practitioners of acupuncture lean towards a more conventional neurophysical explanation, at least in the case of analgesia, which is by far the most widely studied application (Marcus, 1992; Ulett, 1992). I share the view of Quickenden and Tilbury (1986, p. 98) that 'Whether physiologically verifiable effects of acupuncture require any explanation other than direct effects on the nervous system has yet to be shown'.

Perhaps the largest and best equipped enterprise devoted to the objective detection of subtle electromagnetic or other fields around the body was the Dove Project set up by Julian Kenyon in Southampton in 1987 (Kenyon, 1989). This project used sophisticated detection equipment in collaboration with the Department of Physics at Southampton University to investigate such phenomena as Kirlian photography and the use of the Delaware camera and Reich's Orgone Box, devices that in the past have apparently provided evidence in support of 'unconventional' energies associated with the human body in conditions of health or disease.

The Dove Project did detect a persistent luminescence of very low energy (20–130 photons per second) emitted by the body. Nonetheless, in 1989 Kenyon declared that 'so far the light we are seeing from the body does not appear to be anything to do with chi, prana, or the subtle bodies as in the aura'. I am aware of no publications from the Dove Project confirming any aspect of subtle energy since that time. If any positive findings have emerged, they may not have been published because they could be the subject of patent applications (Kenyon, personal communication, 1995). Clearly, it would be of enormous interest to those concerned with subtle energetics to know what, if anything, has emerged from the use of such expensive and highly sophisticated technology.

If such findings have been sparse and unconvincing it may be because calculations by Taylor and Balanovski (1979) of conventional electromagnetic (EM) or other radiations from the human body showed that their power output is very low. But they were not sympathetic to the frequently made claim that so far science has failed to discover the appropriate mechanisms for these phenomena, which nonetheless are valid and remain to be discovered. Such a view was expressed by Hodges and Schofield (1995, p. 205) in relation to the practice of healing: 'observation and practice strongly suggest that the energies associated with healing may be outside the known electro-magnetic spectrum and thus at present unrecognised by science'. For Taylor and Balanovski this appeal to a scientific future is unconvincing: 'there is no reason to support the common claim that there still may be some scientific explanation which has as yet been undiscovered. The successful reductionist approach of science rules out such a possibility except by utilisation of energies impossible to be available to the human body by a factor of billions' (Taylor and Balanovski, 1979, p. 633).

HOW WOULD DEMONSTRATING THE VITAL FORCE INFLUENCE COMPLEMENTARY PRACTICE?

Having considered the evidence for the existence of subtle energy fields, and speculations on the nature of such subtle energy, it is clear that claims for an instrumentally demonstrable state of subtle energy are unconvincing. In the view of Taylor and Balanovski (1979) this is not because we lack the appropriate instrumentation – in addition to the orthodox voltmeter some yet to be developed 'subtle voltmeter' may be required.

However, beyond these questions of whether a subtle energy is demonstrable or not, one issue of fundamental importance remains which relates directly to the *practice* of complementary therapies as opposed to the theoretical bases on which they are said to be founded. The issue is this: what would be the consequence for complementary procedures if a subtle energy were indeed shown to underlie the physical fabric; and conversely what would be the practical consequences if it were not?

The answer to the first question is straightforward. If a bioenergy were demonstrated to exist, practitioners who currently use the bioenergetic model would simply continue to do so and continue to obtain the results that they currently obtain. For example, therapists using 'energy balancing' systems like the *Mora* and *Indumed*, 'which interact with the electromagnetic resonance in the body [with the result that] many totally therapy resistant cases can be treated successfully within three to ten months' (Kenyon, 1987, p. 14) would continue to use them, now with some justification. If notions of *qi* flowing in defined meridians were shown to be valid, then acupuncturists would continue to rebalance it in the way that they always have. And all of those other therapists whose work also depends on energetic balance would continue practising procedures which they knew all along to be well founded.

The more interesting question is what if the concept of subtle energy as a phenomenon that is potentially demonstrable with some appropriate instrumentation were shown to be without any objective foundation? How would that influence complementary practice? Ironically enough, I suggest that the answer is 'hardly at all'. This is partly because few practitioners, convinced by the results of their day-to-day practice, would accept that the notion of subtle energy could ever be invalidated. For most it would be 'business as usual', however difficult it became for them to sustain the subtle energetic model.

The second and more basic reason why the notion of vital energy is likely to persist, whatever the results of enterprises such as the Dove Project to demonstrate it instrumentally, is that it provides a valuable metaphor which is likely to facilitate the success of any therapeutic contact with a complementary practitioner. Our own recent research has centred on what we take to be the purely subjective experiences of *vigour* and *vitality*. We have shown that subjective perceptions of energy can be reliably measured using visual analogue scales and that these perceptions correlate closely with measures of positive affect (Wood and Magnello, 1992). Perceptions of mental and physical energy can also be significantly boosted by short periods of stretching and yogic breathing (*pranayama*) as compared with periods of simple relaxation (Wood, 1993b). At one level this could be regarded as demonstrating an increase in *prana*, a boost in the vital energy of those individuals who practise the appropriate yogic exercises.

However, we make no such claim. We view the perception of vitality as a purely subjective experience. It represents the integration at an affective level of a large amount of physiological information about the body's current capacity to function, information of which the individual is not otherwise aware. The fact that such information is processed via the hypothalamus makes it likely that the actual experience of vigour will be mediated by the limbic system and hence will come to consciousness as an emotional perception rather than an initially cognitive one. Hence, in asking our subjects, 'What is your level of vigour at this moment?', we might equally well have asked, 'What is your level of vital energy?' and achieved a similar answer.

Thus, the subtle or vital energy may be seen as an externalised construct, a reification of an affective or emotional perception. When used for therapeutic purposes this construct provides a shared model for the complementary therapist and for the client who is being treated. The model they share is one of a form of energy which, though not measurable by instruments, both believe to have become depleted or unbalanced. It can be restored by whichever approach (e.g. needles, electrodes or the laying on of hands) the particular therapist is using. The fact that the two do share such a mutually credible model of health and illness is of the greatest importance for the success of the therapeutic relationship and may account for much of the non-specific effects of the treatment.

This 'objectivisation' of subjective experience may be therapeutically valuable but it does nothing to bring the languages of conventional and complementary medicine closer together. For those whose training is in conventional physics and medicine, who are concerned with the measurement of matter and energy and their interconvertability by the living organism, the question of whether the body is surrounded and interpenetrated by a more subtle energetic substance is of fundamental theoretical importance though they conclude that the answer is negative. For the complementary therapist whose procedures are based on a belief in the life force, success depends on that belief, but not on any instrumental demonstration of its reality. This very lack of any need to demonstrate the subtle energy body in order to achieve therapeutic success may give comfort to the therapist's client, whose only desire is to be healed. Unfortunately, does not aid discourse between conventional and complementary medicine.

REFERENCES

Brennan, B.A. (1987) *Hands of Light*, Bantam, New York.
Chopra, D. (1991) *Perfect Health*, Random House, New York.
Glazewski, J.B. (1989) A working hypothesis that defines the complicated nature of Qi. *British Journal of Acupuncture*, **12**(2), 24–5.
Hodges, R.D. and Schofield, A.M. (1995) Is spiritual healing a valid and effective therapy? *Journal of the Royal Society of Medicine*, **88**, 203–7.
Jacobs, S. (1989) A philosophy of energy. *Holistic Medicine*, **4**(2), 95–111.
Kenyon, J. (1987) 'Tuning in' to subtle energies. *Journal of Alternative and Complementary Medicine*, (October), 14.
Kenyon, J. (1989) The Dove Project. *Holistic Medicine*, **4**, 81–94.
Kenyon, J. (1994) Bio-energetic regulatory medicine. *International Journal of Alternative and Complementary Medicine*, (January), 21–5.
LaTourelle, J. (1992) *Thorson's Introductory Guide to Kinesiology*, HarperCollins, London.
Leary, B. (1990) Is vitalism vital? *British Homoeopathic Journal*, **79**, 114–16.
Leskowitz, E. (1992) Life energy and Western medicine: a reappraisal. *Advances: Journal of Mind–Body Health*, **8**(1), 63–7.
Marcus, P. (1992) Acupuncture in modern medicine. *Acupuncture in Medicine*, **10** (Suppl.), 101–8.
Pines, M. (1990) Psychological aspects of energy. *Holistic Medicine*, **5**(1), 5–16.
Quickenden, T.I. and Tilbury, R.N. (1986) A critical examination of the bioplasma hypothesis. *Physiological Chemistry and Physics and Medical NMR*, **18**, 89–101.
Ryman, D. (1984) *The Aromatherapy Handbook*, E.W. Daniel, Saffron Walden.
Schreeve, C. (1988) The subtle truth about energy. *Journal of Alternative and Complementary Medicine*, (December), 17–29.

Seem, M. and Kaplan, J. *Body–Mind Energetics*, Thorsons Publishers, Wellingborough.

Sui, C.K. (1990) *Pranic Healing*, S. Weiser, York, Beach ME.

Tansley, D. (1986) Energy man, energy medicine. *Journal of Alternative Medicine*, (January), 5–7.

Taylor, J.G. and Balanovski, E. (1979) Is there any scientific explanation of the paranormal? *Nature*, **279**, 631–3.

Tisserand, R. (1977) *The Art of Aromatherapy*, E.W. Daniel, Saffron Walden.

Ulett, G.A. (1992) The myth of meridian therapy. *Biological Psychiatry*, **31**, 750–1.

Wood, C. (1986) The body electric in Britain. *Advances: Journal of the Institute for the Advancement of Health*, **3**(2), 56–61.

Wood, C. (1989) The physical nature of energy in the human organism. *Holistic Medicine*, **4**(2), 63–6.

Wood, C. (1993a) Acupuncture, chi and a credible model for treatment. *Acupuncture in Medicine*, **11**(2), 90–4.

Wood, C. (1993b) Mood change and perceptions of vitality: a comparison of the effects of relaxation, visualization and yoga. *Journal of the Royal Society of Medicine*, **86**, 254–8.

Wood, C. and Magnello M.E. (1992) Diurnal changes in perceptions of energy and mood. *Journal of the Royal Society of Medicine*, **85**, 191–4.

Wu, D.Z. (1990) Acupuncture and neurophysiology. *Clinical Neurology and Neurosurgery*, **92**, 13–25.

9

Osteopathy: physiotherapist with time or the practitioner with healing hands?

Stephen Tyreman

INTRODUCTION

Osteopathy in the UK is a profession with an identity crisis. Having spent the best part of 100 years on the fringes of health care provision and in the shadow of conventional medicine, it has found itself suddenly accepted by an establishment previously sceptical about its claims and even hostile to its right to practise. The rapidity of the turnabout, I contend, has left the osteopathic community in a dilemma about whether it is a branch of modern medicine drawing sustenance from scientific medical research and focusing on disease as the explanation of illness, or an autonomous profession rooted in its own unique traditions.

In this chapter, I argue that the osteopaths' drive for professionalisation has progressed on three fronts – political, educational and clinical – and that each in its own way is concerned with identifying the theoretical basis of osteopathy. This is a direct response to the clinical interest shown in osteopathy and other complementary health care systems by conventional medicine, together with decisions about health care policy and the validation and regulation of educational standards in a much broader setting than osteopathy has been used to.

The chapter explores how political, educational and clinical decisions are responding to the challenge of medical interest and scrutiny. Political negotiations seek to identify a niche for osteopathy within UK health care provision; education explores what osteopaths understand to be happening when they encounter clinical problems in the context of broader fields of knowledge;

clinicians explain and attempt to rectify health problems from an osteopathic perspective in the context of a medical model. I contend that osteopathy needs to provide an account of itself in terms that are accessible and open to scrutiny by the public, academia and other health care practitioners. This involves differentiating and describing the normative and descriptive facets of osteopathic theory and practice, in order to analyse them philosophically and scientifically.

OSTEOPATHY AND THE MEDICAL MODEL

What is osteopathy's current relationship with the conventional medical and health care professions and how should it seek to develop them? Should it identify and build on common belief systems, accepting, for example, verification through scientific validation – i.e. by 'independent' scientists outside the profession – or should it look to its non-conformist roots, emphasise its distinctiveness and keep aloof of currently accepted wisdom in the hope that by following what it perceives to be the truth, the tide will turn and medicine will take a form with which osteopathy can identify? In particular, should osteopathy re-examine and incorporate ideas and practices currently ignored and disapproved of by conventional medicine? The founder of osteopathy, Andrew Taylor Still, for example, treated infectious diseases and blindness and a whole range of other conditions. The treatment of back problems barely features in his accounts; for Still, osteopathy was a complete system of medicine which he originally believed would provide an alternative to conventional medicine. To go down this road would involve osteopathy distancing itself from the minor orthopaedic emphasis that characterises much of modern osteopathic practice and which brings approval from conventional medicine.

The medicalisation of osteopathy is a dilemma for patients as much as for practitioners; arguably, as Robin Kirk pointed out in an editorial in the *British Osteopathic Journal*, osteopathy is attractive to some patients because it is different from and offers an alternative to conventional medicine (Kirk, 1995). How might such people react to the professionalisation and new status of osteopathy?

Political decisions

The dilemma over whether or not osteopathy is 'medical' was evident during the long run-up to the King's Fund Report on osteopathy and the passage of the Osteopaths Bill through Parliament in 1993. The General Council and Register of Osteopaths (GCRO), who were the driving force behind the Bill, were fastidious in ensuring that all references to osteopathy in published material emphasised the conventional nature of modern practice and focused primarily on the treatment of musculoskeletal disorders. This was to the chagrin of some members of the profession, who saw it as a lost opportunity to claim that osteopathy could be effective in the treatment of a wide range of conditions from asthma to dysmenorrhoea.

The tightrope walk taken by the professional body had on one side the danger of people concluding that osteopathy is no different from, say, physiotherapy and therefore that there is no justification for granting autonomy, and on the other of people concluding that because it is different and assumes knowledge and concepts unrecognisable to and unacknowledged by conventional medicine, it must lie outside conventional medicine. If it is broadly within the conventional scientific arena, how is it distinctive, and if it offers something new or different, how is this to be incorporated within the conventional body of knowledge?

The question has been largely fudged, in my opinion, by the suggestion being given that what we do can be explained in conventional physiological language, but that there is some extra ingredient in the form of 'manual treatment in which a caring approach to the patient and attention to individual needs are particularly important. In particular, it is concerned with the inter-relationship between the structure of the body and the way in which it functions and is therefore an appropriate form of therapy for many problems affecting the neuro-musculo-skeletal systems.' (General Council and Register of Osteopaths, 1995). Although this is an attempt to communicate a complex concept in just a few words, a cynic might conclude from this statement that an osteopath is a physical therapist who has time to listen to and smile at his or her patient.

Neither is the emphasis on the structure–function relationship a distinctive mark of osteopathy (Tyreman, 1992a): it is an obvious mechanical principle that the structure of a part influences how it works; surgeons, for example, naturally make this assumption. So if osteopathic efficacy is to be explained in terms of the medical model plus some extra ingredient, either the extra ingredient must be defined more convincingly – for example, in terms of vitalism – or the assumption must be re-examined.

The safe ground, to which most arguments justifying the future existence of osteopathy return, is some form of statement to the effect that 'osteopathy works'. Three-quarters of a million treatments are given by osteopaths each year and the small amount of research done suggests that on the whole, patients consider treatment to be effective (Pringle and Tyreman, 1993). Politically, this is not a convincing argument if osteopaths are to maintain independence. Chiropractors and physiotherapists are also effective (though perhaps in slightly different fields) and in these days of interprofessional collaboration in health care, surely it makes more sense to lump all the physical therapies together in one profession and encourage the development of specialisms. There are examples where organisations have taken exactly this approach. In 1993, the Grampian Health Board identified complementary medicine as an area for potential investment and organised a consensus development conference to investigate the possibility of incorporating complementary therapies into NHS care provision (Wilson *et al.*, 1996). With respect to those professions offering manual therapy treatment, they concluded that it was not possible to distinguish between osteopathy, physiotherapy and chiropractic on the grounds of either theory or practice. Unless a good argument can be put forward by osteopaths for why merging with other manual therapists would result in the loss of some significant aspect of patient care, an amalgamation of these professions seems an inevitable outcome.

To date, the main strengths of osteopathy are seen by those outside the profession to lie in the time and attention that can be given to patients – an advantage that may evaporate when or if more osteopathic care is administered under the NHS – and in the palpation and manual skills utilised by osteopaths (General Council and Register of Osteopaths, 1993). These skills, while undoubtedly a hallmark of osteopathy, have yet to be described in terms that can be communicated unambiguously to other practitioners. The difficulty in describing skills was what led Still to impress basic principles on his students rather than techniques. At the present time the claim that osteopaths can detect subtle changes in tissues in a way that is reliably diagnostic is responded to with some incredulity by doctors. When doctors and other manual therapists ask to be taught osteopathic diagnostic and treatment techniques, the response from osteopaths in the past has been to refuse on the grounds that techniques without guiding principles, i.e. acting without thinking like an osteopath, will devalue osteopathy, and only osteopaths can think like osteopaths. So long as this aspect of practice remains a jealously guarded secret, the profession cannot be surprised if those outside do not take it seriously.

Politically, osteopathy has to decide whether it is part of conventional medical care, with the attendant risk that it will become absorbed into a bigger professional grouping, or offer something distinctive, with the risk that it may remain on the fringes of conventional health care. Progress along the middle road – for osteopathy to be integrated into the conventional system while offering a distinctive approach to care – will depend on whether the profession has a loud or clear enough voice in a large and noisy health care arena.

OSTEOPATHIC EDUCATION

The osteopathic educational institutions have faced the dilemma of whether or how to conform to the conventional medical explanatory model for a much longer period of time. The drive for professionalisation and recognition was fought with varying degrees of success in the educational arena before reaching prominence in the political one. The validating process for the British School of Osteopathy's (BSO) BSc degree course by the Council for National Academic Awards (CNAA) in 1988 focused in large part on the scientific credibility of the proposed course. The members of the validating body wanted to be reassured that the school was teaching unsubstantiated dogma. The successful outcome of the validation ironically led to the claim from some in the profession that the BSO had sold its osteopathic birthright for the sake of gaining a validated degree (for a review of the development process, see Edwards, 1990).

The question for osteopathic education is: can the distinctive nature of osteopathy be taught and explored within the context of conventional conceptions of health and illness? If it can, how is it to be done while still maintaining the distinctive nature of osteopathy; and if not, what context will provide the most appropriate setting for describing and communicating the essence of osteopathic care?

In 1992, an internal survey of BSO students soon to graduate, revealed confusion about the emphases on 'medical' and 'osteopathic' approaches to treating patients (Dowdney and Adams, unpublished information). Students felt that the distinctive osteopathic emphasis behind explanations and management of clinical problems was being squeezed by the medical orthodoxy coming into the teaching of medical practice subjects. In other words, osteopathy had an interesting theory behind it, but it was difficult, or perhaps politically impractical, to put into practice.

OSTEOPATHIC CLINICAL PRACTICE

The dilemma for clinical practice is linked to the educational debate and focuses on the relationship between diagnosis and treatment. In the inaugural issue of the *British Osteopathic Journal*, Colin Dove, arguably one of the chief architects of modern osteopathy, published a paper entitled 'The place of medical diagnosis in clinical osteopathy' (Dove, 1960). He argued that osteopathy was not and could not be an alternative system competing with conventional medicine. In his view, diagnosis has to combine osteopathic structural examination with conventional clinical methods. He approached the problem from the standpoint of 'missed pathologies', i.e. that traditional osteopathic musculoskeletal evaluation cannot reveal all the pathological states that can threaten the health of a person. Osteopathy therefore has to 'borrow' conventional diagnostic techniques in order to recognise certain diseases. But while this solves the problem of failing to diagnose and treat pernicious illnesses, it appears to exaggerate the division between osteopathic and conventional medical explanations; perhaps it puts them in a complementary relationship, but nevertheless ultimately it separates them as different from each other in some fundamental way. This may not be a problem – psychological and physical diagnoses appear to exist reasonably comfortably together in conventional medicine without using a common foundation – but because osteopathy and medicine both claim to be evaluating physical states of health, it seems that some common ground should be identifiable. Although this has been achieved to some extent – Irvin Korr, for example, has described the sympathetic nervous system as providing an organising link between the musculoskeletal system and the visceral organs (Korr, 1979) – a clear conceptual framework has still to be developed.

Most health care disciplines have a clear, conceptual basis to their diagnosis and treatment: in medicine, a practitioner may identify a deficiency in a chemical such as insulin and replace it; a surgeon may remove abnormal or potentially harmful tissue; anti-inflammatory drugs are given to counteract inflammation and so on. The diagnosis leads logically to the prescription of the most appropriate treatment. Physiotherapy has developed within this tradition: exercises are given to build up lost muscle strength; mobility is improved through stretching, heat improves blood flow in hypertonic muscle; and ice is used to reduce inflammation. In each case, the diagnosis points to the appropriate treatment because there is a common conceptual model underlying diagnosis and treatment. This is not so obviously true for osteopathy.

During the 1970s osteopathy underwent a radical change when the long-held concepts of 'osteopathic lesions', illness as the result of deviations from ideal mechanical states, and complex diagnostic analyses of relationships between key areas of the body, were replaced by more medical explanations of tissue and pathology (for an overview, see Hawkins, 1985; Smith, 1985). The focus was the identification of local tissue states causally responsible for the symptoms and the illness. Audrey Smith, another of the chief architects of modern osteopathy, referred to this analytical method as a 'pathological sieve' because the process involved reducing the components of the lesion into its constituent parts based upon a knowledge of the local anatomy and physiology. This diagnostic scheme consisted of examining the standing, sitting and recumbent patient, using a combination of observation and palpation, then from a sound knowledge of anatomy, physiology and pathology, normal and abnormal tissue states could be deduced.

This scheme responded to the practical problem Dove had identified, in that it brought osteopathic examination techniques to bear on conventional patho-physiological conceptions of tissue states. It was simple in its basic conception – utilising accepted anatomical, physiological and pathological principles – while remaining open enough to encompass a broad view of the patient. However, it suffered from two fundamental problems. First, it was primarily reductionist, whereas the osteopathic instinct is to consider the person in his or her wholeness. This would not be a problem if putting the parts together again to present a different, clinically useful picture was an integral part of the method, but the scheme never developed that far. What was needed was a system that was primarily holistic while encompassing methodological reductionism. The failure to achieve this may have led directly to the ambiguity in students' minds referred to above over the extent to which osteopathic theory and practice is an adjunct to conventional medicine or something distinct.

The second problem is a clinical one: by describing lesion states in terms of their anatomical and pathological components, diagnosis is separated conceptually from traditional osteopathic technique. For example, if a medial collateral ligament of the knee is diagnosed as inflamed, traditional osteopathic technique has no anti-inflammatory procedures to counteract it; the same is true for diagnosis of, say, a herniated or prolapsed intervertebral disc. This is not to suggest that osteopathic techniques cannot effectively change these states, only that there is no obvious common concept to link diagnosis with treatment logically. With the more traditional diagnostic approach, an osteopath diagnosing a vertebral segment as, say, fixed in flexion relative to its contiguous segments would employ a technique to encourage extension; a joint with a limited range of movement can (in theory) have that range increased with the appropriate technique. But once the lesioned state is analysed in terms of tissues and pathologies rather than mechanical principles, it leaves standard osteopathic technique isolated. An inflamed ligament cannot be explained in mechanical terms of leverage, force, direction, velocity and so on, though of course the pathological state might have mechanical consequences.

It appears that this dilemma has only two solutions: either osteopathic explanations must become prescriptive on the basis of empirical data – pathological tissue state X requires techniques A,B and C – or it must restate its conceptual explanation in terms that are common both to diagnosis and treatment or in some way link them. The prescriptive option has been anathema to osteopaths; it is claimed (perhaps piously) that osteopaths are concerned with people and whole illnesses not syndromes and conditions. To practise osteopathy in terms of states requiring set prescribed treatments would be to go against deeply held beliefs. This leaves the necessity to link mechanical with physiological concepts, or to restate the theoretical basis of diagnosis and treatment, though these tasks are not necessarily mutually exclusive. However, to date, neither task has been cogently attempted.

This highlights the central need for critical research in osteopathy, which must, I believe, consist of a two-pronged approach – philosophical and scientific. Normative, philosophical research will inquire into the conceptual basis of osteopathic care by examining osteopathic explanations of health, illness, disease and care, while scientific research will examine mechanisms and correlate clinical data. Both further highlight the dilemma in the extent to which osteopathy might adopt a broadly medical model both to explain (philosophical), and to validate (scientific) its practice.

Research in osteopathy

The questions implicit in the choice (or not) of whether to adopt the medical model in research methodology cannot be separated from questions emerging from the educational and clinical arena. At the present time there is no clear picture emerging of the direction research might take.

The result of philosophical analysis may determine the focus for scientific research. For example, if diseases are considered to be real entities that are most effectively explained and treated by detailed investigation into their pathology, aetiology and specific characteristics, then the function of research is to uncover as much of that kind of information as possible. On the other hand, if disease is considered to be a nominalistic concept – it just happens to be useful to categorise particular states as diseases in order to identify and treat (potentially) threatening events – then research will focus on explaining and identifying what the circumstances are that produce those states. To take tuberculosis (TB) as an example: the medical model approach to research focuses on identifying the disease, tuberculosis – what its symptom pattern is, pathological changes, aetiology, prognosis and so on. But a different approach would be to examine those states that make TB such an undesirable human condition by perhaps focusing on hygiene, immune responses, social conditions and those factors that permit such a state to develop. According to this view, TB may be thought of as an altered physiological state which is life threatening, undesirable or inappropriate rather than a discrete entity ontologically different from 'normal' physiological states.

The focus on diseases is a fundamental part of the medical model, though theorists in the philosophy of medicine and health care are beginning to question how valid it is in the context of modern epidemiological patterns of illness and disease (see, for example, Engel, 1977; Fulford, 1996; Gabe, Kelleher and Williams, 1994; Greaves, 1979; Nordenfelt, 1995; Seedhouse, 1991). More holistic or anthropomorphic health care focuses on factors associated with and necessary for the development of unfavourable health states, including the patient's own beliefs and expectations about the illness. While each approach may be equally valid in terms of providing effective health care, each requires a different scientific method to investigate it. As osteopathy becomes more involved in researching its practice, these differences will emerge as significant pointers in the development of a valid osteopathic research model.

The dilemma over whether osteopathy is essentially conventional, accepting the prevailing beliefs and mores of the medical model, or comes from a different set of beliefs will form a focus for debate over the next few years as the profession establishes itself in the public health care arena. It is not a problem unique to osteopathy, or even to complementary and alternative health care. The relationship between science and medicine and the extent to which science is an appropriate validating discipline is again a live issue (Delkeskamp-Hayes and Gardell Cutter 1993; Forstrom, 1977; Foss, 1989; Gatens-Robinson, 1986; Greaves, 1979; Tyreman, 1992b).

USING 'PRINCIPLES' TO GUIDE OSTEOPATHIC DECISION MAKING

It was suggested earlier that Andrew Taylor Still, the founder of osteopathy, found it difficult to communicate the treatment and diagnostic skills associated with osteopathy to his students. Instead he impressed certain 'principles' on to them in the belief that by applying these natural, 'God-given' principles to individual clinical situations, students could work out for themselves what the most appropriate diagnosis and treatment were. Still's classical triad of principles, 'structure governs function', 'the rule of the artery is supreme' and 'the body contains its own medicine chest' are generally acknowledged to lie somewhere near the heart of osteopathic practice. But to what extent do they either define osteopathic care, or guide clinical decision-making?

Structure governs function

Still's understanding of the relationship between the body's ability to function properly and effectively and the structural integrity of body parts is both complex and subtle. That there is a causal link between a structure and its function is uncontroversial. What is interesting in the principle, is the use of the verb 'governs' to describe the link between structure and function, because 'govern' can mean 'rule or control', 'influence or determine' or 'be a standard or principle for' (Allen, 1990). In addition, 'govern' can mean 'define the boundaries of' in the sense that in a democratic society, for example, a government lays down laws that effectively define what is not permitted and by implication (and common law) allow people freedom to act within those boundaries. In this sense, structure could be interpreted as the parameters that determine functional range. For example, structural degeneration in a hip joint has implications for the function of that joint because it limits the range of movement.

We do not have any way of knowing for certain which of those meanings Still intended – if he was sure himself. He does not provide us with any clear definition of either structure or function. We can try to interpret what he might have meant in the light of his and other contemporary writings, but we will have an interpretation rather than a defining principle.

The rule of the artery is supreme

This is an even more problematic statement. The use of 'rule' and 'supreme' to describe circulation is somewhat bizarre. If, as is frequently assumed, Still intended to convey the idea that an efficient blood supply is important for the healthy functioning of body tissues, this too is uncontroversial, but is perhaps a modern interpretation of Still. If he was claiming something more than this – for example, that all disease is the result of impaired or inadequate blood supply, which in the light of his writing would be a valid reading – that is more contentious and a conclusion with which many practitioners would feel uncomfortable.

The body contains its own medicine chest

This was a most astute perception coming as it did before medical understanding of the immune system, but it is hardly a guide to treatment. Knowing that the body is capable of self-correction and homeostatic balance does not tell a practitioner what to do in a certain case, only that the body, in a particular but unspecified state, has the capability of correcting itself. Still assumed that if the body parts were properly arranged, i.e., if the structure was sound, then access to the 'medicine chest' was automatically gained and the body's innate healing systems would counter the disease process. This hints at serendipity rather than planned treatment with anticipated specific outcomes. If true, if it is possible to release endogenous chemicals to counteract specific diseases, then much more research is necessary to demonstrate the relationship between treatment and such physiological responses. If not, if it is indeed a question of doing certain things to the body and expecting a favourable physiological effect, then that too must be explained as an alternative to the medical model.

These principles are interesting and arguably provide a basis for understanding and developing what Still understood osteopathy to be. However, they do not provide a firm enough set of guidelines on their own to allow a practitioner to make decisions about what information is relevant or what treatment will be effective. If principles are to provide a practical guide for osteopaths, they must be applicable in identified circumstances and suggest a particular course of action.

MODERN RESTATEMENTS OF STILL'S PRINCIPLES

At various times in the history of the profession there has been an attempt to re-evaluate and restate what is unique or distinctive about osteopathy. Perhaps the most widely accepted set of criteria was defined in the USA over a 30-year period beginning in 1953. It can be seen how the ideas have evolved from the original intuition of Still. The eight precepts are set out as follows:

(1) The body is a unit.
(2) Structure and function are reciprocally interrelated.
(3) The body possesses self-regulatory mechanisms.
(4) The body has the inherent capacity to defend and repair itself.
(5) When normal adaptability is disrupted, or when environmental changes overcome the body's capacity for self-maintenance, disease may ensue.
(6) Movement of body fluids is essential to the maintenance of health.
(7) The nerves play a crucial part in controlling the fluids of the body.
(8) There are somatic components to disease that are not only manifestations of disease but also factors that contribute to maintenance of the diseased state (Martinke, 1991).

At first sight these statements appear to compensate for the inadequacies of the original triad: they are less ambiguous, more explicit and as explanations of the body operating in health and illness, use common physiological language. The problem is that neither individually nor collectively are they unique to osteopathy. The list could probably be used to describe just about any health care profession – conventional or complementary.

The other problem with the eight precepts is that they fail to capture the subtlety of Still's intuitive understanding of body health and illness. There is a feeling that the list is trying to interpret Still in the light of the medical model, restating mysteries in down-to-earth biological language. What it does provide however, is a description of the broad outlook of osteopathic care – the ethos. Reading those tenets gives the practitioner coming from a conventional medical background a feel for the general approach and understanding of osteopathy.

AN ALTERNATIVE APPROACH

Irvin Korr, an American physiologist long associated with osteopathic research, outlined the function of the autonomic nervous system, in particular the sympathetic component, in a series of papers (Korr, 1970, 1979). He noted that the autonomic nervous system in general and the sympathetic branch in particular lay between the visceral and somatic body components (the word 'somatic' is used here in a technical sense to include all musculoskeletal structures and connective tissues, rather in the literal sense of 'body structure'). He suggested that the division of visceral from musculoskeletal body elements made sense if conceptualised in terms of the actions of the person. So-called visceral structures function to support and maintain the musculoskeletal system. He argued that people value the ability to act, to move, to do things, rather than how their livers, kidneys or hearts function. If they do value the latter, it is only because medicine teaches that kidneys and livers make a vital contribution to human activities, but this is a rationalised rather than an intuitive association.

If this conceptualisation is correct then the musculoskeletal system can be considered to be the body machinery through which a person acts. Korr referred to this as the 'primary machinery of life' and argued that everything about human existence that is regarded as valuable is ultimately expressed through the musculoskeletal system. Even philosophy and religion are only valuable to the extent that they change or influence behaviour, or can be communicated. If it cannot be expressed in some form, it is not valued. Human life therefore, is primarily concerned with action.

If this model is extrapolated further, there are some interesting implications. The concept of function is seen to consist of a purposeful hierarchy of body properties whose ultimate goal is the implementation of activity. The function of the heart is to pump blood rather than to make a sound, or occupy space – others of its properties – because pumping blood (among other things) allows muscles to operate and the person to do things. The evaluation of how effectively or efficiently a particular body part is functioning is with reference to the extent to which it is effective in contributing to the activity of the person. The value afforded to this activity is negotiated and agreed between patient and practitioner and acknowledges personal expectations, physiological limitations, social mores and so on.

From this kind of analysis, Lennart Nordenfelt has concluded that health is related to the ability to pursue and achieve goals, (1995) and Bill Fulford has concluded that illness is therefore 'action failure' (1989). This overturns the usual assumption that illness is explained by disease (Boorse, 1975; Scadding, 1988) by saying that illness is a state of health whose reality is agreed between patient and practitioner. Because this particular state interferes with the patient's ability to perform certain actions (according to agreed norms of ability and comfort), it therefore constitutes a state of affairs requiring medical attention. Physiology as the study of function is thus seen to be a second-order description of action. Physiology, according to this account, is the scientific, biological description of function, i.e., those body processes contributing to the person's ability to act, or countering those environmental forces that might interfere with action.

Traditionally, osteopathy has focused on assessing and treating the musculoskeletal system. As a therapy, it should be ideally placed to evaluate function at first hand in terms of the actions of a person. It has a number of advantages over health care systems based on other concepts of illness: it operates closer to the basic function-informing values – the actions of the musculoskeletal structures themselves – rather than through physiological values which are necessarily one stage removed from their informing sources. I say 'should' because at the moment osteopaths do not appear to have developed a sufficiently sophisticated explanatory account of what they do in practice. This, I contend, is due to the ambiguity about osteopathy's association with the prevailing medical model. It should be possible, for example, to develop a diagnostic approach that focuses on actions rather than pathologies. What does walking do to the psoas muscle, the liver and the trapezius? How do these very different kinds of body parts relate to each other to allow a person to walk normally?

Bevis Nathan has described how a systems understanding of the body can enable osteopaths to consider the leg, the thorax and the abdomen as systems, instead of thinking in terms of the musculoskeletal, cardiovascular or respiratory systems, which he describes as classes of tissues (Nathan, 1994). It should be possible to develop this kind of approach in the direction of thinking about a person's actions and the ways in which specific body parts are involved. This in turn may begin to provide more effective accounts of why particular body tissues and organs become vulnerable to disease.

This approach is not new, it has been part of the osteopath's intuition since Still, though it has not always been well taught or practised. What the profession has lacked has been a coherent theoretical account on a par with the scientifically validated medical model; which brings us right back to the original dilemma – osteopathy has yet to decide whether it should offer an alternative to the medical model, or find its niche among other health care disciplines by integrating with that model.

CONCLUDING COMMENTS

In this paper I have not commented on the suitability of the medical model for conventional medicine, only pointed out the model's deficiencies and shortcomings when applied to osteopathy. Osteopathy's strength, and perhaps its distinctiveness, lies in its focus on the structural and functional integrity of the musculoskeletal system rather than on diseases or illness syndromes. I have argued that, because health care practice and theory require a common conceptual base, the medical model with its focus on disease is not applicable to osteopathy unless it abandons its traditional clinical territory and becomes aligned, say, with physiotherapy. It follows therefore that if osteopathy is to continue as a distinctive, autonomous profession, it must find an alternative model to describe its particular way of thinking and working. I have suggested that because the concepts of function and dysfunction appear to lie at the heart of osteopathic thinking, they will form vital elements in any analysis and eventual defining account of osteopathy. However, no such account of exactly what function is has been articulated.

REFERENCES

Allen, R.E. (ed.) (1990) *The Concise Oxford Dictionary*, 8th edn, Oxford University Press, Oxford.

Boorse, C. (1975) On the distinction between disease and illness. *Philosophy and Public Affairs*, **5**, 49–68.

Delkeskamp-Hayes, C. and Gardell Cutter, M.A. (eds). (1993) *Science, Technology, and the Art of Medicine*, Kluwer Academic, Dordrecht.

Dove, C.I. (1960) The place of medical diagnosis in clinical osteopathy. *British Osteopathic Journal*, **1**(1), 1–13.

Edwards, D. (1990) The development of a course in osteopathy in the UK. *Complementary Medical Research*, **4**(1), 32–45.

Engel, G.L. (1977) The need for a new medical model: a challenge for biomedicine. *Science*, **196**, 129–36.

Forstrom, L.A. (1977) The scientific autonomy of clinical medicine. *Journal of Medicine and Philosophy*, **2**(1), 8–19.

Foss, L. (1989) The challenge to biomedicine: a foundations perspective. *The Journal of Medicine and Philosophy*, **14**(2), 165–91.

Fulford, K.W.M. (1989) *Moral Theory and Medical Practice*, Cambridge University Press, Cambridge.

Fulford, K.W.M. (1996) Concepts of disease and the meaning of patient-centred care, in *Essential Practice in Patient-Centred Care* (eds K.M. Fulford, S. Ersser and R.A. Hope), Blackwell Science, Oxford, pp. 1–16.

Gabe, J., Kelleher, D. and Williams, G. (eds), (1994) *Challenging Medicine*, Routledge, London.

Gatens-Robinson, E. (1986) Clinical judgement and the rationality of the human sciences. *Journal of Medicine and Philosophy*, **11**(2), 167–78.

General Council and Register of Osteopaths (1993) *Competences Required for Osteopathic Practice*, GCRO, Reading.

General Council and Register of Osteopaths (1995) *Osteopathy: The Facts*, GCRO, Reading.

Greaves, D. (1979) What is medicine? Towards a philosophical approach. *Journal of Medical Ethics*, **5**(1), 29–32.

Hawkins, P.J. (1985) *A Textbook of Osteopathic Diagnosis*, Tamor Pierston Publishers, London.

Kirk, R. (1995) Editorial. *British Osteopathic Journal*, **17**, 3–5.

Korr, I.M. (1970) The sympathetic nervous system as mediator between the somatic and supportive processes, in *The Physiologic Basis of Osteopathic Medicine*, (ed. J. Buzzel), Postgraduate Institute of Osteopathic Medicine and Surgery, pp. 21–38.

Korr, I.M. (1979) The spinal cord as an organiser of disease processes: the peripheral nervous system. *Journal of the American Osteopathic Association*, **79**, 82–90.

Martinke, D.J. (1991) The philosophy of osteopathic medicine. *An Osteopathic Approach to Diagnosis and Treatment* (eds E.L. DiGiovanna and S. Schiowitz), J.B. Lippincott Company, New York & London, pp. 3–6.

Nathan, B. (1994) Philosophical notes on osteopathic theory. *British Osteopathic Journal*, **13**, 8–15.

Nordenfelt, L. (1995) *On the Nature of Health: An Action-Theoretic Approach*, 2nd edn, D. Reidel Publishing Co., Dordrecht.

Pringle, M. and Tyreman, S. (1993) Study of 500 patients attending an osteopathic practice. *British Journal of General Practice*, **43**, 15–18.

Scadding, J.G. (1988) Health and disease: what can medicine do for philosophy? *Journal of Medical Ethics*, **14**, 118–24.

Seedhouse, D. (1991) *Liberating Medicine*, John Wiley & Sons, Chichester.

Smith, A.E. (1985) A survey of the osteopathic diagnostic method, in *A Textbook of Osteopathic Diagnosis* (ed. P.J. Hawkins), Tamor Pierston, London, pp. 11–24.

Tyreman, S.J. (1992a) Concepts for osteopathic health care. *Journal of Osteopathic Education*, **2**(1), 10–17.

Tyreman, S.J. (1992b) Orthodox and heterodox medical philosophy: a comparative study. MA dissertation, University of Wales.

Wilson, B.J., Goodwin, N., Grimshaw, J.M. *et al.* (1996) Complementary therapies in a local healthcare setting. Part 2: an experiment in bringing complementary therapies into local NHS commissioning. The Grampian Consensus Development Conference. *Complementary Therapies in Medicine*, **4**(2), 118–23.

<table>
<tr><td>10</td><td># Is complementary medicine holistic?</td></tr>
</table>

10	# Is complementary medicine holistic?

David Peters

INTRODUCTION

This chapter investigates whether complementary medicine is holistic. One approach might be to compare a set of 'holistic principles' with the theory and practice of complementary/alternative medicine (CAM). But this would perhaps be to ignore the limitations of language, its inevitable inaccuracy, how words depend on their context for meaning. The word 'holistic' has several meanings, depending on the context in which it is used. In order to understand the question: 'Is CAM holistic?', we need to understand what we mean by 'CAM' and 'holistic'. To do this, we must explore the social, cultural and historical background of contemporary health care. We will not be able to understand the implications of holism, nor make sense of our current medical predicament and 'complementarity' without taking into account what I will call 'Modernity's crisis of visions and values'.

How CAM implies and expresses holism will be explored here along with its lack of reflexivity – that is, its failure to apply its principles to itself – and for its confusing use of language. The overall theme will be how CAM can be seen as a 'signpost' for important changes in our health beliefs.

MODERNISM AND MEDICINE

To understand the recent interest in CAM and holism, it would be helpful to make reference to concepts used in socio-cultural commentary and critique. Two terms that are frequently used to discuss current or recent aspects of culture are 'modernism' and 'post-modernism'. Modernism can be described as a set of beliefs, generally implicit, that scientific understanding will increase our technological control of the world. Such control often takes the form of dramatic intervention – transplant surgery or large-scale engineering projects would be good examples – and is thought to lead to human progress in terms of increased happiness and well-being. Generally speaking, modernism favours a single way of explaining the world.

Post-modernism starts from the position that the world cannot be understood in terms of a single framework. Understanding comes from examining and juxtaposing multiple perspectives and from accepting a disjointed plurality of values and beliefs. As such, post-modernism is deeply suspicious of the assumption that progress is implicit in technological advance.

Conventional medicine is often described as 'biomedicine' because it emphasises the link between medical intervention (technology) and biological understanding (science). As such, conventional medicine is a modernist enterprise. Critics of biomedicine might make great play of its failure to address chronic degenerative and malignant disease, and of the problem of iatrogenesis, that is, ill-health caused by medical treatment. But biomedicine is perceived as unsatisfactory for another, less specific, reason, namely a distrust of modernity. For although biomedical perspectives are enormously valuable, they cannot incorporate a number of late twentieth century aspirations and concerns about a variety of issues: the purpose of life, the body as a whole, the question of responsibility for illness, personal agency in promoting health and the meaning of disease.

Holism can be interpreted as a response to what could be identified as the 'crisis of representation' in biomedicine. This means that the images and metaphors used by biomedicine to explain the world have come into question. Take, for instance, the image of the person as a biological machine, or the concept of inexorable progress, absolute scientific truth and medical infallibility. These apparently key representations of biomedicine are widely disputed, hence, a 'crisis' of representation.

Biomedicine has produced awesome technical achievements, yet it provides no 'stories to live by'. The belief that dramatic intervention is the answer to medical problems has become as unsustainable as medical utopianism and omnipotence. The human genome project, as a symbol for the next giant leap for biomedicine, is a good example. Ambivalence about the project's ambition and nightmarish eugenic possibilities is a characteristic experience for those suspicious of the modernist enterprise.

CAM is well-placed to benefit from recent cultural shifts away from modernity because of its post-modernist outlook. Common themes in CAM which may be described as post-modernist include the incorporation of traditional and indigenous perspectives alongside the scientific language of psychology, biochemistry and sociology; the fragmentation of knowledge into disjointed parts; a distrust that science and technology will bring unproblematic progress. It appears to offer new ways of representing health and of addressing those concerns which seem to have been left outside biomedicine.

As such, the rhetoric that CAM is a holistic answer to the problems of contemporary medicine can seem natural, even obvious. It is this 'natural and obvious' that I seek to examine in the remainder of this essay. In order to do so, I will analyse some common beliefs about CAM and holism.

CAM AND HOLISM: SOME COMMON BELIEFS EXPLORED

The wider availability of CAM would make the population more healthy by preventing disease

Significant areas of conventional medicine are dedicated to improving the health of populations: there is an associated class of doctor (public health) and of medical research (epidemiology). Generally speaking, there is good evidence for much of conventional preventive medicine, be it clean water, cervical screening or advice to stop smoking. Conversely, there is little or no evidence that CAM can improve the long-term health of populations. Despite this, a supposed ability to prevent disease is a common feature of CAM rhetoric.

Why should the idea of CAM as preventative medicine have developed? One explanation is that, sometime, new ideas about the world emerge which influence individuals and set cultural change in motion. There are those who say holism is just such an idea and that it heralds a new paradigm. The inevitable subtext – of a new order (of healthcare) offering redemption (from the ills of materialist civilisation) by repentance (paradigm shift) and right conduct (change of beliefs and lifestyle) – seems inescapable, especially now that the language of 'health', 'wholeness' and 'holiness' have become so hard to extricate. However, the dangers of this quasi-religious approach should be obvious.

CAM can cure what conventional medicine cannot: and can do so without side effects

If the rise of CAM is, in part, a response to biomedicine's broken promises of cure, then we should be suspicious of claims that it provides another set of technical fixes. More particularly, the problem with any claim that a particular therapy is effective and safe is that practitioners of all types make such claims. CAM practitioners may 'know' their treatments work (after all, they see their patients get better) and they may even cite the massive popularity of CAM as evidence. However, presumably exactly the same thing might be said by proponents of unusual surgical techniques such as gastric freezing, or by those obstetricians who continue to give women medically unnecessary caesarean sections.

There are, no doubt, significant problems in CAM research. One of the most intractable is whether (and how) to distinguish the effects of therapist and therapy. But this argument has been misrepresented by a few practitioners to back their assertion that research is altogether a wasted effort. I would argue that cost- and risk-benefit are important issues and that research into effectiveness and safety need to go hand in hand whatever the treatment. The claim that 'CAM can cure what conventional medicine cannot' should not be made without strong evidence to that effect.

CAM treatments can address the 'real causes' of disease

CAM practitioners often use depth metaphors. Homoeopaths may attribute disease to 'miasms' (long-term inherited traits), the after effects of emotional trauma or even spiritual causes. Naturopathy's explanatory model implicates accumulating 'toxins', and treats chronic inflammatory disease by encouraging 'detoxification' via the bowel, liver, kidneys and skin. Traditional Chinese Medicine (TCM) views disease such as eczema as either a failure of the liver to organise metabolic processes, as a disorder of assimilation, or of inadequate elimination.

It is entirely possible that though homoeopathic, naturopathic and TCM theory is couched in language unfamiliar to biomedicine, further research will show them to be worthwhile pragmatic models for treatment. Even if this were to be the case, depth metaphors would remain just that, metaphors. It is problematic for a practitioner to refer to an apparently metaphorical cause (such as miasms) whilst treating a disease and then use the success of treatment as evidence for the reality of the metaphor. To claim that CAM treatments address the real causes of disease, CAM practitioners would need to demonstrate the reality (however interpreted) of the causes they claim are related to ill-heath.

CAM unifies mind and body, and is able to treat the body through soul and spirit

When it claims insight into psychological causes of disease CAM often seems simplistic, prescriptive, atheoretical and overly-reliant on the poorly articulated insights of charismatic founder figures. For example, Louise Hay tells how negative attitudes transform into specific diseases; a notion superficially akin to Franz Alexander's more developed concept of psychosomatic illnesses – he includes rheumatoid arthritis, ulcerative colitis and peptic ulcer – which he linked to psychological types, (but unlike Hay he offered no specific affirmations to treat them). Alexander identified a mere seven types; Bach flower remedy aficionados find 39 underlying emotional causes, each one having an associated flower essence. Rebirthers take a different psychological slant; implicating traumatic birth events which predispose us to disease, they believe that re-experiencing these can promote better health.

The question of whether any of these versions of mind–body unity has practical value becomes more complicated when CAM intermingles with new approaches to psychotherapy, with 'personal growth' and with practical spiritual traditions deriving from the East. This is an understandable cross-fertilisation and it arises for two main reasons: firstly, spiritual practice – meditation, yoga, Qi gong – is entangled in the roots of traditional oriental medical systems and is only partly separable from them; secondly, CAM shares a common language set with aspects of humanistic psychology which are concerned with consciousness, the meaning of experience, the transformation and harmony of thought, feeling and action.

The result of this cross-fertilisation between CAM and psycho-spiritual practices, the 'New Health Culture' as it has been termed, is problematic. Its protagonists see it as the illuminating context which turns non-conventional therapies into keys to personal growth and levers for social transformation and cultural change. Others say it confuses debate about new and possibly useful therapies by surrounding them with superstition and mysticism. Moreover, the 'New Health Culture' can be individualistic, psychologically naive and apolitical. It can play a quasi-religious function, turn health into a commodity and implicitly denigrate those who fail to overcome illness.

CAM can explain and name what conventional medicine cannot

Can a CAM diagnosis be of value by constructing a diagnosis which enables therapeutic leverage where conventional medicine has none? Or are such labels misleading?

Take, for example, a woman experiencing persistent fatigue who consults a CAM practitioner. A naturopath might diagnose magnesium deficiency, a hidden allergy to food or 'dysbiosis' (involving a failure of detoxification processes, acquired gut hyper-permeability and alterations in bowel flora). An osteopath might suggest structural-behavioural causes such as a breathing dysfunction. An osteopath interested in cranial techniques, on the other hand, might diagnose a problem with the 'primary rhythm' of cerebro-spinal fluid circulation. A homoeopath might invoke miasms or constitutional disturbance. An acupuncturist would suggest organic processes were at fault (such as deficient Spleen *chi* following an invasion of Wind), unless, perhaps, he or she was of a 'five elements' orientation, in which case diagnosis would be biased towards more symbolic-psychological explanations (such as an excess of Metal, perhaps implying an obsessional trait or psychological inflexibility). A herbal medical practitioner would aim to determine the balance and vitality of different organic processes, particularly digestion, circulation and elimination. The patient might also visit a health show and obtain a diagnosis of 'geopathic stress'; malign electro-magnetic influence due to domestic electrical circuitry, local transmission equipment, underground water currents, disordered Feng Shui or Ley lines.

Such diagnoses are only of benefit if they enable better coping, curing or caring or if they promote insight and make an experience meaningful. Has this been shown to be the case? Or is it possible that a CAM diagnosis might hinder effective copying or curing, for example, by encouraging dietary change when diet does not have an important effect on the presenting illness? And could a CAM diagnosis lessen insight, for example, by attributing a physical cause, such as electromagnetic radiation, to a problem which is primarily psychological? In short, even if CAM can explain and name what conventional medicine cannot, this is not necessarily a good thing.

CAM diagnosis is holistic

With its central metaphor of comprehending disease as the outcome of dysfunctional processes potentially involving the whole person – CAM represents a counter-balance to biomedicine's passionate focus on confronting established pathological change at ever more microscopic levels. CAM generally conceives of the body and mind as a single informational entity; often giving a central role to energy as an explanatory basis for aetiology and treatment. Diagnosis generally involves looking at the patient in context; relies largely on the patient's own account of their experience and views the patient as having agency and choices.

Yet the previous examples of some typical diagnoses include highly reductionist explanations. In reaching their diagnosis different practitioners use diverse methods: some mechanical and recognisably scientific, others apparently paranormal. Nutritional testing, for instance, sometimes employs conventional laboratory methods. Practitioners may also base diagnoses on pendulums, Kirlian cameras, and various electrical tests, more or less computerised, to identify relevant homoeopathic medicines, food supplements and allergies.

Generally CAM avoids hi-tech diagnosis in favour of using hand and eye, guided by unconventional theory. Most homoeopaths base their prescriptions on an extensive history of symptoms (though some use a computer to analyse these symptom complexes and match them to the toxicology of their remedies). TCM acupuncturists usually diagnose from history, pulse and tongue appearance, though a few use electrical point locators, or even complex computer applications to detect channels and organ disorders. If CAM can include reductionist and mechanistic elements, use synthetic medicines and incorporate fragments of technology then the case for its being inherently 'holistic' or 'natural' is not a straightforward one.

CAM offers more humane care

CAM practitioners have a reputation for being more caring than their conventional counterparts. It might be argued that this results from biomedicine's pursuit of active ingredients to cure 'real' diseases, something which does not do much to encourage professionals to act humanely or engage with their patients any more than is necessary for completing a technical task. Yet conventional healthcare – especially in the sphere of nursing – recognises that time, touch and generating a therapeutic relationship are important. On further consideration, it seems implausible that the sorts of people who enter training schools in say, osteopathy, are more caring than those who choose a medical training. More likely, it is under-resourced systems of health-care delivery which put a strain on practitioners and dampen their ability to relate to clients. The social phenomenon of CAM might give conventional practitioners cause to reflect on the way in which they offer care to patients. Doctors who have trained in CAM, for example, often report improved clinical skills as a result. Nonetheless, it is difficult to support any argument that CAM is inherently more humane than conventional medicine.

Even if CAM does have a capacity to promote humane, patient-centred, process-oriented, psychosomatic, empowering approaches to therapy, it must also be said that this is not a unique feature of CAM. Moreover, even though these approaches may satisfy significant post-modern needs, and enhance the therapeutic alliance, this does not necessarily entail that CAM's ideas about aetiology, diagnostics and the technical aspects of treatment are authentic.

CAM approaches the body as a whole

There is a tension between my body as I experience it and my body as it is experienced and interpreted by another. Compare, for example, an individual patient's experience of pain and a conventional diagnosis of osteoarthritis, described in terms of hidden changes to the physical structure of hidden tissue. Though CAM does not always deal directly with the patient's subjective experience of illness, its descriptions of health seem closer to everyday experience than those of psychotherapy or physiotherapy, let alone anatomy or pathology.

This is an important clue about why CAM is so popular: it may be fulfilling the need for a post-reductionist, non-mechanistic approach to the body. But one expression of this new approach to the body is the eclectic symbol-mix labeled 'New Age' thought. At its most naive, it is a collision of ancient and recent notions where the magical, the miraculous, the spiritual are equated with anything else beyond ordinary understanding, including hyper-modern science (especially quantum physics or holography) and the esoteric (commonly Theosophical interpretations of Eastern thought). The New Age seems to take these ideas and their overlapping metaphors literally, speaking of 'the New Paradigm' or 'holism' and 'energy' as though they were concrete realities. But they are not explanatory terms; rather they reveal holes in our imagination which can only be filled with meaning if we use the ideas tentatively, bearing in mind that they signify something dimly understood.

POST-MODERN HEALTH CARE: COLLABORATION AND INTEGRATION?

One of CAM's undoubted strengths is its capacity to generate powerful beliefs and expectations in practitioners and clients. If in the future mainstream medicine reclaims these non-specific processes – which it presently marginalises and brackets off as mere placebo effects – it will be largely because CAM, and research into CAM, has made it impossible to ignore their importance. CAM profoundly blurs all the distinction which biomedicine has so carefully constructed: between subjective experience and objective reality; mind and body; practitioner and patient; therapy and therapist; the modern and the medieval.

CAM is an expression of post-modernity; and though it is a signpost for holistic post-modern medicine, I think it is not the destination. Problems arise if CAM is represented as a 'New Order' of health care; an alternative; a triumphalist anti-scientific movement; a set of easy answers. If understood dogmatically and literally, CAM can be misleading and potentially repressive. It can also be described as atavistic, that is, incorporating elements of that which is outdated and has no place in the contemporary world. CAM practitioners often seem to treat ideas as if they were facts, give metaphors (such as the meridian system) a place in the physical world and are guilty of magical thinking: the conviction that believing something necessarily makes it so. They contrast their holistic approach with a stereotype of conventional medicine when under-resourced and practised in its most extreme biomedical form and thus present their aspirations as though they were antithetical to the values and practices of mainstream care.

Moreover, it may be holistic (and appropriately post-modern) to juxtapose psychological, biochemical and sociological language sets with indigenous and traditional standpoints. But it can also be very confusing if these language games generate a kind of 'magical holism'. The craving for inclusiveness can become yet another big story in itself. Is it holistic to be incomplete? In a sense we are, for aspects of human incompleteness are timeless: vulnerability, limitation, dependency; the need to make hard choices and tolerate imperfection. The Modernity project's agenda was to abolish them all through rational scientific progress: 'magical holism' prefers simply to deny them. They are different kinds of defence against uncertainty and incompleteness.

It would be too easy to reject CAM for this lack of sophistication if this were all there was to it. I have tried to explain why I believe CAM is not inherently holistic; though in the theories and practices of CAM, aspects of a holistic approach are reflected. Nor can CAM hope to stand still any longer as if cocooned in a medieval and magical world-view where it might once have been protected from the scientific gaze in whose unsubtle glare it now stands. For it is already engaging with mainstream culture in universities, hospitals and laboratories; it is responding to the challenge of the biopsychosocial approach. Mature CAM practitioners have a growing compassion for the state of conventional medicine and a deepening understanding that the uncertainty and vulnerability of professional life is something they share with conventional practitioners. At their best, CAM and evolving biopsychosocial medicine seem to be striving in the same direction; and a rapprochement between highly developed non-western systems and biopsychosocial medicine seems all the more likely as post-modern healthcare evolves to include subjective experience and a patient-centred approach. A wish to collaborate in education, practice and research, therefore, seems inevitable. It remains to be seen how a vitalistic CAM and a biopsychosocial medicine can re-shape one another. If this can be achieved while retaining what is best in biomedicine, we will have achieved one step towards an integrated, post-modern and holistic health care.

FURTHER READING

Foucault, M. (1976) *The Birth of the Clinic: An Archeology of Medical Perception*, Tavistock, London.

Illich, I. (1976) *Limits to Medicine. Medical Nemesis: The Expropriation of Health*, Pelikan, London.

Engel, G. (1977) The need for a new medical model: the challenge for biomedicine. *Science*, **196**, 129–36.

Coward, R. (1989) *The Whole Truth: The Myth of Alternative Health*, Faber and Faber, London.

Watkins, A. (1997) *A Practitioner's Handbook of Mind–Body Medicine*, Churchill-Livingstone, Edinburgh.

A critique of assumptions made about complementary medicine

11

Anthony Campbell

INTRODUCTION

In this article I will critique some of the philosophical assumptions that contribute to the popularity of complementary medicine.

ASSUMPTION 1: COMPLEMENTARY MEDICINE IS NATURAL

This is probably the single most important claim made on behalf of complementary medicine. A large number of patients who come for treatment give this as their reason. Yet the concept of the 'natural' is by no means clear-cut. We can distinguish at least the following components.

(1) In the case of herbalism and homoeopathy the important consideration is the origin of the medicines. These are typically derived from vegetable or (in the case of homoeopathy) mineral or animal sources, and they are usually used whole, i.e. the complete plant or animal is used to make the starting solution. This is in contrast to conventional pharmacology, where even if the medicines are not wholly synthetic they are isolates of an active principle. Homoeopaths and herbalists claim that using the whole of the source material is advantageous because the various constituents act together in a balanced manner. Even within orthodox medicine the use of whole plant extracts died out only quite recently: as late as the 1960s some of the older physicians were still using digitalis (foxglove) leaf tablets to treat heart failure in preference to tablets containing just the active ingredient, digoxin.

(2)   The idea of the natural is not applied only to medicines. Acupuncture and other hands-on forms of treatment are also accorded the accolade of 'natural'. This may seem a little odd – after all, there is nothing very natural about needling people – but the underlying idea is that these treatments make use of the innate healing capabilities of the body. Orthodox treatment, in contrast, is supposed to take no account of these capabilities or even actively to damage them.

(3)   A closely related idea is that the natural state of the body is one of health, and that illness results from an imbalance of some kind (often described as an 'energy imbalance'). An inference that is very commonly drawn from this supposition is an optimistic view of symptoms. For orthodox medicine symptoms are a clue to the underlying pathological process. Once they have enabled a diagnosis to be reached they serve no useful purpose and should be relieved if possible, even if the disease itself cannot be cured. In complementary medicine, in contrast, there is a widespread belief that symptoms represent the healing process at work and should therefore not be suppressed. This attitude entails an important consequence: the symptoms are endowed with meaning. No longer are discomfort, pain and weakness things to be endured with whatever degree of stoicism one can muster; rather they should be viewed in a positive light because they represent the wisdom of the body. It is often said that disease will get worse before it gets better when the right treatment is given, an idea that is particularly ingrained in homoeopathy, where it originated with Hahnemann's doctrine of the homoeopathic aggravation.

If we look critically at these assumptions we find that the concept of the natural in complementary medicine is questionable from a number of points of view. The comforting belief that 'natural' somehow equates with 'safe' is manifestly mistaken. The natural world abounds with toxins; indeed it would be hard to match in the laboratory the toxicity of naturally occurring compounds like ricin or the poison of the deathcap mushroom. Bacteria and viruses are natural too. The fact that a herbal medicine is 'natural' by no means guarantees its safety. Critics have often made this point, but there is another, perhaps more fundamental, flaw in the assumption that 'natural' equals 'desirable'. This assumption is based on a misapprehension about what the world of nature is really like. Much that is written about complementary medicine seems to assume a benevolent Mother Nature, who acts as a protectress, provided we don't transgress her rules. But nature can also be pictured as Kali, dancing naked on the bodies of her victims and wearing a necklace of human skulls. Perhaps, we ought to regard her as simply indifferent, at least to the survival of the individual.

It is an inevitable feature of a competitive system, which is what natural selection is, that there should be losers as well as winners. For a variety of reasons some individuals will find themselves less than optimally adapted to their situation, and much disease results from such maladaptation. Again, evolution is concerned to ensure reproduction; once the individual has successfully reproduced, his or her role is largely finished. True, at the human level there may have been some selective advantage in having parents and other relatives live long enough to pass on some of their cultural knowledge to the next generation, but this is unlikely to have favoured survival much beyond the age of about 45. If we take the idea of 'the natural' seriously, therefore, we should recognise that our present increased life span is in a sense unnatural, and it is hardly surprising that, as we age, degenerative and malignant disease become more and more frequent. Especially where older patients are concerned, optimistic statements that the body is essentially healthy are destined to encounter harsh biological realities that give the lie to such comforting beliefs.

To pursue the question of why we should be so impressed today by the alleged virtues of the natural would be too great a digression, but we should note that this attitude is relatively modern. When homoeopathy began, in the early nineteenth century, little was said about its being natural. What seems to have happened is that, as science and technology have advanced and more and more of us have adopted an urban lifestyle, we have come to have an increasingly romantic, not to say sentimental, view of nature. In recent years this tendency has been enhanced by a flood of television documentaries representing the natural world less as a scene of conflict and mayhem and more as a kind of ecological cooperative where all would proceed in blessed peace and harmony were it not for the disruption introduced into this idyllic scene by the ever-growing menace of human intervention, which disrupts the harmony of nature in a dozen ways: pollution, global warming, deforestation, extinction of species – the list grows constantly. Just as we insensitively damage the environment in pursuit of short-term aims, so on the inner, physiological level we try to bulldoze our way to health using powerful drugs. But though these may seem to work at first, they cannot promote real lasting health because they are 'against nature'.

The concept of the natural, then, is a powerful myth which works at many levels and it is not surprising that it should be so influential in complementary medicine. It is nevertheless based upon misapprehension and sloppy thinking.

ASSUMPTION 2: COMPLEMENTARY MEDICINE IS TRADITIONAL

Modern technological medicine is a recent development and, perhaps as a reaction, most forms of complementary medicine make a point of claiming to be ancient or traditional. Some forms of complementary medicine are indeed ancient. Acupuncture certainly falls into this category and so do some other oriental imports such as Ayurvedic medicine, even though in many cases there has been a good deal of relatively recent elaboration and reinterpretation. Although the origins of the treatment may be lost in the mists of time, there is often a more or less mythical personage who is credited with inventing or discovering it; in the case of acupuncture, this is the legendary Yellow Emperor. Other forms of therapy, such as homoeopathy, chiropractic, osteopathy or the Alexander technique, being of more recent origin, can point to a real founding father (or sometimes mother), although this personage is often represented as having revived some long-lost traditional knowledge. Samuel Hahnemann, for instance, claimed to have found anticipations of homoeopathy as far back as Hippocrates (although he curiously omitted to include the much more relevant figure of Paracelsus among his intellectual forebears). Thus the founder is usually at once innovator and traditionalist.

Founders are almost always credited with possessing near-superhuman wisdom and insight. Much of the argument that goes on within the ranks of complementary practitioners centres on the recorded utterances of these heroes, almost as if they were scriptural documents. Sometimes the mantle of the originator of the system becomes draped, after his death, on the shoulders of a later disciple, and this process may continue on down the generations. This is particularly evident in homoeopathy, where for many homoeopaths, even today, the nineteenth-century figure of James Tyler Kent has acquired almost the authority of Hahnemann himself. As a result we hear about 'classic homoeopathy', which is really Kentian homoeopathy; few of its advocates seem to realise that in his own day Kent was considered something of an interloper and that his version of homoeopathy owes a good deal both to the Swedish mystic Emanuel Swedenborg and to the system of medicine, called Eclecticism, in which Kent was originally trained (Wood, 1996). Present-day epigoni continue the tradition. It is not difficult to think of modern practitioners in many branches of complementary medicine who have built up considerable followings among pupils who accept their gurus' pronouncements unquestioningly and proselytise for them with enthusiasm.

The founders of complementary medical systems are often credited with having discovered, or rediscovered, eternal truths. Hahnemann believed that he had done this and his successors down to the present echo that claim. Thus we are told that homoeopathy is founded on 'the basic laws of healing that, while they have always operated and are valid for all ages, have only in modern times been discovered and formulated in systematic fashion' (Vithoulkas, 1980). This is an attempt to be simultaneously old and new. The important thing to notice about such claims is that, whatever one's opinion of their validity, they are contrary to the principle of scientific inquiry. They hark back to mediaeval reliance on authority (Aristotelian and Galenic pronouncements), whereas science is forward looking and iconoclastic. This brings us to the question of authority in complementary medicine; as so often in this area, we are confronted by paradox.

ASSUMPTION 3: COMPLEMENTARY MEDICINE IS ANTI-AUTHORITARIAN

To what extent is complementary medicine anti-authoritarian? In some ways it could be regarded as a reaction against the 'power' of the medical profession, and it is often represented in this light. To the extent that it constitutes such a reaction it is in tune with much contemporary thinking, and not only within medicine: all authority figures today are suspect. The expression 'doctor's orders', which used to be heard a lot forty or fifty years ago, may not have disappeared completely, but it is certainly much less common today. The notion of the doctor as the expert who must be deferred to is becoming unfashionable, and instead we are encouraged to take responsibility for our own health, and to view the doctor as a co-worker in the enterprise rather than an authority figure. Not all doctors, it has to be said, welcome this trend, though some do. In theory, complementary medicine is supposed to encourage patient participation in making decisions, but there often seems to be a tendency for the complementary therapist to take on the role of the expert which the doctor is supposed to have abandoned. And patients usually go along with this – which is hardly surprising, for unless you regard a therapist as an expert in their field, what is the point of asking their opinion?

A recent survey of complementary practitioners in the British Midlands, carried out by Ursula M. Sharma, then of the Centre for Medical Social Anthropology at the University of Keele, investigated this question among others. Dr Sharma found that, although the therapists she interviewed generally believed in treating the patient as an individual and expected her or him to be an active partner in treatment, they were also pulled in the other direction by their wish to be more 'professional' and to lay claim to genuine forms of specialised knowledge. As Dr Sharma remarks, 'The practice of non-orthodox medicine abounds in contradictions, some internal and others imposed from outside.' (1991.)

The founding fathers and mothers of complementary medical systems have nearly always been strongly authoritarian. Hahnemann, for example, would tolerate no deviation on the part of his disciples and referred contemptuously to those who combined homoeopathy with allopathy as 'half-homoeopaths'. When one of his closest disciples, who had had the misfortune to lose a child, remarked that the experience had taught him that homoeopathy was not the answer to everything, Hahnemann was furious and never fully restored him to favour. When a homoeopathic hospital was established in Leipzig, Hahnemann, by now living at Kothen, took exception to the medical director on the grounds that he was not sufficiently committed to homoeopathy, and had him replaced; unfortunately the new director soon left and his successor, who bore the appropriate name of Fickel, took the job with the undeclared aim of discrediting homoeopathy, and the ensuing débâcle led to the closure of the hospital.

The later homoeopath J.T. Kent was also an uncompromising authoritarian. Thus he wrote, 'It is law that governs the world and not matters of opinion or hypothesis. We must begin by having a respect for law, for we have no starting point unless we base our propositions on law. So long as we recognise men's statements we are in a state of change, for men and hypotheses change. Let us acknowledge the authority' (1932). But whose authority are we to acknowledge? Presumably Hahnemann's; but surely Hahnemann was a man, and therefore no more exempt from error than other men? Not so, Kent implies, for Hahnemann had discovered a divinely ordained law. Homoeopathy is an inspired science, which is the only true kind of science; all the rest is mere opinion. It is therefore not merely foolish but actually impious to question Hahnemann. By implication it is also impious to question Kent. There are similarities here with Freud: psychoanalysis has many of the features characteristic of a complementary medical system.

ASSUMPTION 4: COMPLEMENTARY MEDICINE DEALS WITH CAUSES

One of the oddest features of complementary medicine concerns the idea of cause. Many patients say, 'I don't want to take a drug just to suppress my symptoms, I want to find the cause.' This idea is prevalent in complementary medicine: we constantly see claims that conventional medicine merely deals with the manifestations of disease instead of eradicating it at the root. Interestingly, many conventional practitioners say the exact opposite.

The explanation is that the two groups have different ideas of what constitutes a cause. For orthodox medicine 'cause' contains the idea of pathology. A disease may be due to a parasite, a genetic factor or an environmental toxin, for example, but in all cases the ideal explanation will include an account at a molecular level of what has gone wrong and how the phenomena of the disease – the symptoms – are produced. Complementary medicine, in contrast, is comparatively uninterested in such questions. True, there is a certain amount of overlap between the two: orthodox medicine today pays increasing attention to the role of the environment and of lifestyle in the production of disease, whereas complementary medicine has produced its own theories of disease which include roles for supposed infections. For example, the candida theory implies that all kinds of symptoms are due to a chronic overgrowth of candida in the intestine, and the role of viruses is central to much theorising about ME. This is an old idea in complementary medicine; Hahnemann's miasm theory of chronic disease is best understood as an early attempt to account for long-lasting symptoms in terms of chronic infection (Campbell, 1984). But in such cases there is little interest in offering detailed accounts of how the putative infection actually causes the symptoms in question; it is enough to state that they do. These 'pathological' theories in complementary medicine are not really capable of offering serious explanations of disease; they are more like what the late Richard Feynman called 'cargo cult science' – they have the superficial character of scientific theories but lack genuine scientific content.

There is considerable enthusiasm in complementary medicine for psychological explanations of disease. Some attention has been paid within orthodox medicine to so-called psychosomatic disorders but the role of the psyche is greater for complementary practitioners. This reflects a considerable, and largely unrecognised, shift in the readiness of patients to accept that psychological factors may play a part in causing the symptoms of which they complain. Some ten or twenty years ago suggestions to this effect were usually unwelcome, but today few patients object to the notion that 'stress', that universal and amorphous modern bugbear, has played a role in precipitating whatever it is they are complaining of.

Causation theories in complementary medicine have psychological advantages from the point of view of many patients. First, they are relatively easy to understand. Molecular medicine and modern genetics are difficult subjects even for professionals and they cannot easily be made comprehensible at a popular level. Second, even if they can be understood they are not necessarily very meaningful at a human level. Many patients ask, either explicitly or implicitly, 'why me?', and this is as much an existential question as a pathological or scientific one. The kind of answer that complementary medicine offers – the illness has occurred because of something that has happened to you in the course of your life, or because you have adopted a faulty pattern of thinking or feeling or reacting to life, or have been eating the wrong foods – is seen as meaningful by many people. Moreover, and this is important, it tends to carry optimistic connotations. You cannot do much about a molecular disorder, except perhaps at an advanced technological level, but you can certainly alter your diet or even your whole lifestyle.

A third reason why the diagnoses commonly offered by complementary medicine practitioners are popular is that they are pronounced confidently and provide the patient with a label for their disease. A conventional doctor may well not be able to offer a diagnosis for a patient who complains of numerous ill-defined symptoms that do not fit any definite nosological category. This leaves the patient feeling dissatisfied or even alarmed that some obscure disorder is being missed. A visit to a complementary practitioner may then yield a firm opinion that the problem is due to candida. Receiving a diagnostic label is enough in itself to make many patients feel better.

ASSUMPTION 5: COMPLEMENTARY MEDICINE IS NOT MATERIALISTIC

A powerful, though often unacknowledged, reason for the appeal of complementary medicine is that it is based on a non-materialistic view of human nature. Whereas orthodox medicine is seen as trying to explain everything in mechanistic terms, complementary medicine is perceived as having a more widely based approach. In one survey nearly half of the sample of holistic practitioners replied that religious and spiritual experiences were important in shaping their views about health, illness and healing, in contrast to 13% of family practitioners (Nanke and Canter, 1991). There are many references in the complementary medicine literature to a tripartite model of the human being – body, mind and soul. In conventional medicine, on the other hand, the trend is entirely in the opposite direction, so that psychology itself is increasingly coming to be seen as a branch of neurology, with psychiatric disorders being seen as disorders of the brain, which can and should be investigated as such. This idea may be acceptable to modern psychiatrists (perhaps with a few dissenters) but it is probably not acceptable to the majority of patients. Many of us tend instinctively to be unconscious Cartesian dualists and to picture ourselves as minds inhabiting bodies. This way of thinking is more at home in complementary medicine than in modern technological medicine. Sometimes it is expressed in more or less overtly religious or mystical terms, but sometimes an attempt is made to formulate it in a scientific way, usually drawing on modern quantum physics for an explanatory framework. 'If we are to remain true to science, we must integrate the data that science provides us, and be willing to follow where the process leads. It is increasingly evident that physics requires us to acknowledge metaconsiderations; that is, considerations that lie above and beyond physics. Those of us biomedical practitioners who base our work on physics cannot disparage as "merely metaphysics" a metaphysics to which physics itself points.' (Bessinger, 1996.)

Writers such as Bessinger want to escape from the materialism of modern biology and medicine but without abandoning science altogether, and they hope that they can enlist science itself, in the form of quantum physics, in this cause. Their arguments are expressed at an abstruse philosophical level and do not impinge greatly on the day-to-day work of complementary practitioners. They are probably read by only a small minority of such practitioners who happen to be interested in thinking about the philosophical basis of what they are doing. Nevertheless, the climate of thought in complementary medicine is predominantly sympathetic to ideas of this kind.

CONCLUSION

I have tried to show that the appeal of complementary medicine depends on its philosophical assumptions as well as its practical effects. Inevitably I have had to generalise: there are many forms of complementary medicine, and not all of them, and not all the practitioners within any one form, are equally committed to the ways of thinking I have outlined. Nevertheless I have no doubt that the trend is in the direction I indicate. If this argument is correct it implies that the growth in popularity of complementary medicine is likely to continue, more or less regardless of the outcome of research intended to evaluate the efficacy of the treatments in question. This is because the philosophical basis on which much complementary medicine rests fulfils a psychological need for many people who feel disoriented and lost in a world that seems to leave less and less space for basic human values.

REFERENCES

Bessinger, C.D. Jr (1996) Reflections on reality, healing, and consciousness. *Alternative Therapies*, **2**, 40–5.

Campbell, A. (1984) *The Two Faces of Homoeopathy*, Robert Hale, London, pp. 49–54.

Kent, J.T. (1932) *Lectures on Homoeopathic Materia Medica*, Boericke & Tafel, Philadelphia.

Nanke, L. and Canter D. (1991) Treatment recommendation in complementary medicine: a selective network. *Complementary Medical Research*, **5**, 1–7.

Sharma, U.M. (1991) Complementary practitioners in a Midlands locality. *Complementary Medical Research*, **5**, 12–16.

Vithoulkas, G. (1980) *The Science of Homoeopathy*, Grove Press, New York, p. 3.

Wood, M. (1996) *The Magical Staff: The Vitalist Tradition in Western Medicine*, North Atlantic Books, Berkeley.

PART FOUR

Towards scepticism

This section explores both the origins and possible amelioration of low levels of critical self-analysis in complementary medicine. George Lewith argues that good quality research can help to overcome many debates and difficulties. He points out that both critics and proponents have ignored the research evidence and that many complementary practitioners have condemned traditional research methods because they have failed to understand them. Ursula Sharma's paper looks at a more internal debate within one complementary therapy. She argues that homoeopaths have not developed a critical discourse within which to evaluate knowledge claims. If two homoeopaths disagree, there is no shared method by which to settle the dispute. Maria Hondras explores the links between research and professionalisation in chiropractic. She charts the obstacles of those trying to promote chiropractic research, identifying in particular, the use of empty rhetoric about science ('chiropractic is scientific'), the insistence that 'chiropractic works' and unsound generalisations from poorly understood original research. In conclusion, she argues for the development of an institutional infrastructure to support research and scholarship in chiropractic.

Reasonable consensus, self-criticism and the grounds of debate: a case from homoeopathy

12

Ursula Sharma

INTRODUCTION

In this paper I shall consider the problem of how knowledge is developed and how debates about the best ways to practise health care can be resolved in a professional group that has not yet established a collective tradition of research into efficacy of treatment. To illustrate the problem I shall discuss in some detail the debate about prescribing which erupted among members of the Society of Homoeopaths in 1992. The particulars of this debate are specific to homoeopathy but the issues are of wider relevance in complementary medicine. This is because pertinent features of the homoeopathic profession are similar to those of many other complementary therapies.

A vital component in the development of a modern profession is an agreed body of knowledge, codified to a high degree and transmitted through formal modes of training and education. For knowledge to be codified, the professional community needs to develop a reasonable consensus on principles that can be referred to in case of disagreement, and methods of moderating disputes on fact or theory.

I say 'reasonable consensus' because probably in most professional groups there is only approximate agreement on many matters – enough to prevent frequent schism and enough to define the range of positions and practices that can be accommodated without a total redefinition of the special competence of that profession. Where the accumulation of new knowledge is concerned, the principles also need to be flexible enough to allow for growth and change – but not so flexible that members of the professional community have no common reference points for the evaluation of new ideas or methods.

Complementary therapies are practised in Britain today by a group of emergent professional communities. Some of these have moved further than others towards the state I have just outlined and there is a diversity of political processes through which a workable effective consensus is sought. I shall illustrate some of the problems involved in this process with reference to a particular professional community, that of the non-medically qualified (NMQ) homoeopaths in Britain. In particular I have followed the debates and processes taking place among members of the Society of Homoeopaths, exemplified in their publications, conferences, meetings and other public output.

The Society of Homoeopaths is the larger of the two main professional organisations of NMQ homoeopaths in Britain, having over 400 members. Founded in 1978, it has made impressive progress in developing a common core curriculum for homoeopathic students, rigorous registration procedures, an active ethics committee, high-quality house journals and all the other features of a modern professional body. Much, though by no means all, of what I shall have to say about the Society may also be applicable to members of the United Kingdom Homoeopathic Medical Association (UKHMA) – indeed they have a number of members in common in spite of their rather different historical traditions – but I know less about the UKHMA and am reluctant to generalise.

DEFINING BOUNDARIES: AN INTERNAL DEBATE

In January 1992, Robert Davidson and David Howell, two long-established members of the Society of Homoeopaths, who for some time had been discontented with what they saw as the predominance of a somewhat narrow form of homoeopathy, convened the first meeting of what they called the 'Not Just Classical Club' (NJC). I understand the title of the group to indicate that they saw their methods of prescribing in terms of an addition to the classical form of homoeopathy rather than as something intended to displace it altogether. Nevertheless, the inauguration of this group provoked fierce debate within the Society. Some saw it as a major questioning of that which makes homoeopathy uniquely valuable, while others saw it as a refreshing and enabling departure in the direction of a more practical and beneficial mode of prescribing. What follows is not an exhaustive rehearsal of all the arguments made and justifications provided, only of the kind of terms in which the debate was conducted. This account should illustrate some of the problems the NMQ homoeopathic community faces in developing the 'reasonable consensus on principles' referred to above.

Homoeopathy, whether practised by NMQ homoeopaths or by medical doctors with a training in homoeopathy, is based on the principle that 'like cures like'. Its practice involves the administration of a highly dilute form of a substance that would, in its undiluted form, cause a healthy person to display the very symptoms from which the patient suffers. Ill health is not understood in terms of biomedical disease categories so much as in terms of profiles of symptoms and characteristics such as temperament and taste in food. Much prescribing is described as 'constitutional'. The practitioner attempts to find a remedy that corresponds to the basic constitution of the patient rather than to isolated, often transient symptoms. Much of the professional knowledge of the homoeopath consists of knowledge of the properties of these remedies, how to discover the right remedy for the individual patient and how then to prescribe the remedy with the appropriate potency and timing, when to decide that a different remedy is called for, and so on.

In what has come to be called the 'classical' mode of prescribing, the practitioner holds to the principle of the administration of a single remedy at a time. The classical homoeopath, having thoroughly explored the patient's symptoms and characteristics, decides on a single most appropriate remedy and waits for its effects to manifest themselves before either repeating this remedy or using some other remedy.

On the whole, the Society of Homoeopaths has been regarded as upholding a classical approach to prescribing. In a statement designed to help homoeopaths to explain the principles of their treatment to the public at large, the Society pronounced:

In homoeopathy only one remedy . . . is used at a time. Just as a television reproduces only the programme to which it is tuned, so a sick person is very sensitive to or 'tuned-in to' the correct remedy and only a minute stimulus from the right signal (or remedy) is required. This is sometimes called the principle of the minimum dose.

Society of Homoeopaths (1991, p. 2).

Some NMQ homoeopaths had for long regarded this as excessive purism and had developed combination remedies, where more than one remedy is given at a time, in combination or in quick succession. Those who found the NJC ideas useful claimed that the Society was covertly or openly moving to a dogmatically classical position in which there was no room for the questioning of a fixed orthodoxy. In the face of such accusations, Robin Logan, one of the Society's registrars, was at pains to point out that when representatives of the Society examined the clinical cases submitted by candidates for registration with the Society they did not exclude people with good potential as homoeopaths on the grounds that they prescribed in a manner that was not strictly classical:

I have been a registrar for two and a half years and in that time not a single conscientious homoeopath has been refused on the basis of the

type of cases they have submitted . . . I cannot make up my mind what
is behind such rumours.

But he also stated that

Some patients are prescribed 4 or 5 of these complexes (i.e. complex
remedies) at a time. Where do we draw the line? Is unconditionally
accepting the claims that methods work really what you are suggesting?
You wouldn't believe the range of extraordinary claims that one comes
across in a job like this.

Logan (1992, p. 27)

This statement points to a crucial problem, namely that NMQ homoeopaths do
not have a standardised means of judging and comparing claims of efficacy,
whether submitted by prospective candidates for registration or by established
practitioners. When a homoeopath (or group of homoeopaths) using one
method of prescribing, publicly challenges one who uses a different method,
each can only assert that their method does indeed work and offer accumulated
examples of success (i.e. success as defined by themselves). Hence it was difficult
for either the classicist or the 'not just classicist' to find ways of convincing each
other (or for that matter anyone else) of the superiority of their approach.

SOLVING PROBLEMS AND ADDING TO KNOWLEDGE

Homoeopathy does have a tradition of research, through what its founder
Hahnemann called 'provings'. In a 'proving', a dose of the remedy to be tested
is given to a number of healthy volunteers (usually pupils or associates of the
homoeopath who is conducting the proving) and the entire range of subsequent experiences or symptoms are carefully noted. This has been the way
in which new remedies have been added to the homoeopathic materia medica.
The early proving of snake venom, lachesis, is famous. Recently, Jeremy Sherr
has conducted provings of hydrogen and chocolate.

One of the problems with provings is that they are not designed to be
comparative, or at any rate have not been used in a comparative way in the
past. While some provers do now introduce a placebo with which to compare
the effects of the remedy to be proved, the numbers involved in the trial are
seldom great enough to carry out tests of statistical significance. For example,
in Jeremy Sherr's proving of hydrogen, 18 provers participated, of which three
were given a placebo. No reference is made to the experiences of the provers
who were given the placebo, so no comparison is possible. The results of
provings have not enabled homoeopaths to quantify the effects of a remedy
in such a way that they can compare it with the quantified effects of another
remedy. A proving is better understood as a means of exploring the possible
effects of a new remedy rather than as a means of measuring those effects.

This does not mean that individual homoeopaths do not make comparisons at all. They may well compare the effects of different remedies on individual patients or on a group of patients. An important way in which knowledge is stored and passed on in the homoeopathic community is the convention of the case history, publicly presented at a seminar or in a published article. This will usually take the form of a narrative of how the patient was treated, what remedies were given and what effects they had, and may involve the admission of false starts and errors as well as (usually) a successful conclusion, the homoeopath taking the audience or reader through the process of reasoning used to arrive at an appropriate remedy. To take one example at random, in an article entitled 'A *gratiola* case' Roberto Bianchini describes how he treated a patient who had (among other symptoms) severe eating problems with *cyclamen*, *anacardium*, *medhorrinum* and *pulsatilla* 'with little effect'. He then goes on to describe how through careful attention to the patient's rather dreamy disposition, which he had previously overlooked, and through careful study of well known repertories, he arrived at the remedy gratiola. He then describes how a course of doses of this remedy in ascending potencies brought about a general improvement, albeit interrupted temporarily by the recurrence of some old symptoms. The way this case is presented - in the form of a narrative in which the homocopath describes the way she or he reasoned from the symptoms and the store of available homoeopathic knowledge – is fairly typical (Bianchini, 1994, p.197).

This kind of discourse does not provide a means for the development of standardised criteria for comparison of remedies or methods of prescribing, focusing as it does on the ways in which a particular case or a particular type of case was managed. The main comparison that can be made by the homoe-opath is whether the same patient gets better more or less rapidly under successive regimes, not whether different patients having similar symptoms do better or worse when different remedies or modes of prescribing are used.

MEDIATING DIFFERENCE, EVALUATING SUCCESS

One contributor to the 'classical' / 'not just classical' debate lamented the fact that it was actually difficult to evaluate the evidence for different techniques, since many seminars and master classes at which cases are presented by experienced homoeopaths are too expensive for the ordinary student or practitioner to attend: 'What exactly are people doing? why are they doing it? and what criteria are being used to evaluate success?' (Crockett, 1992, p. 27).

In the absence of an agreed method for collecting and evaluating evidence for the claims of the adherents of different modes of prescribing, it was perhaps inevitable that the debate should be conducted in terms of the consequences of NJC for the profession rather than in terms of the consequences of NJC for patients treated through these methods. Some argued the value of open mind-edness versus ideological orthodoxy: 'Let us build bridges first and talk to each other with open minds' (Crockett, 1992, p. 27). 'If Hahnemann were alive today he would probably be doing something totally different as he was continually updating his methods.' (Harper, 1992, p. 27). Others contributed to the discussion in terms of the consequences of strife and division for the profession:

> We really do need to pull together and stop wasting this energy. After all we should be training each other and training ourselves . . . not only for each other but for the people we treat. Giving love is the most important thing, not the destructive criticism we have at present.
>
> Miles (1992, p. 22)

> The NJC Club . . . has linguistically 'split apart what is already whole' by dividing homoeopathy into 'classical' and 'not just classical'. To my mind there is only one kind of homoeopathy . . . whether homoeopathy is classical or not is irrelevant – homoeopathy is homoeopathy.
>
> Brinkley (1992, p. 28)

Another theme that was taken up was the claim (made by Tony Southam in a leaflet advertising an NJC Club seminar) that by using 'not just classical' methods of prescribing one could cure more people more quickly. This was seized upon by some as welcome news, by others with scepticism. Some feared that this involved a degeneration of homoeopathy from its tradition of highly individualised prescribing. Or was it just unsubstantiated boasting?

> If someone can see and treat 30 patients on a daily basis and 'cure' them in the broadest meaning of the word and not just treat their ailments, then more power to them. If there are strategies and methodologies for doing so why not publish them in an open forum such as this Newsletter or *The Homoeopath* and make them available to a far wider range of practitioners than can be reached in a seminar?
>
> Brinkley (1992, p. 29)

> My contention is that the prescriber who is happy with a 70% success rate and minimal interviews cannot advance their own level of understanding . . . For those of us who aspire to excellence rather than remaining content with a basic level of competence the issue actually does become how to cure 90% of 6 people a day.
>
> Norland (1992, p. 25)

> How can one have affection for 30 patients a day (150 patients a week) i.e. one every fifteen to twenty minutes? I do not believe it is possible and that 'doing what works' means ignoring the character of each individual patient and going for simple recipes or routines.
>
> Chatfield (1992, p. 25)

There was evidently a fear that this manner of prescribing might achieve simple and superficial alleviation of symptoms in the short term without attacking the deep-seated causes of patients' ill health, which is what leads to 'cure' in the long term. The fact that many patents are satisfied with such short-term removal of symptoms, argued the classicists, is neither here nor there.

Tony Southam, originator of the claim, responded that homoeopathy is fun, simple and easy:

> I enjoy enabling people to regain a more acceptable level of health . . .
> To imply that if a practitioner is seeing a lot of patients then they are not curing them is a strange thing to do. Especially as referral by cured and satisfied patients is the way that such a practice creates a consistent volume of new patients. To state that the classical/alchemical practitioner knows much better than the patient what the patient needs is a very strange and perhaps arrogant position. It is certainly an assumption of spiritual superiority.

> Southam (1992, p.27)

I do not mean to suggest that rhetoric and ideological persuasion were the only resources open to NMQ homoeopaths in the conduct of this debate. In a debate reported in the pages of *The Homoeopath* (on the motion 'This house believes that the single remedy is the medicine of experience'), David Curtin defended the single-remedy approach in terms of the logic of the approach rather than in terms of research data. If you give the patient several remedies at once, he argued, they may interfere with one another. If you give a hundred remedies you are likely to hit the simillimum (i.e. the remedy that matches most exactly the patient's profile) by chance, as it were, but you will not have such good results as if you worked to find out the simillimum and gave that alone. His opponent, Dr George Lewith, defending the use of multiple remedies, noted that Curtin's argument amounted to an argument about the single remedy being useful as a means of practitioner learning (rather than in terms of the patient's interest in being cured quickly), and criticised an argument based on a single practitioner's experience (Curtin *et al.*, 1993).

OUT OF THE IMPASSE?

This debate illustrated very clearly an impasse that homoeopaths were experiencing because of the lack of agreed criteria for testing and comparing new practices and ideas. Because there was no agreed way of evaluating outcomes, the debate had to be conducted in terms of 'my experience versus your experience', open-mindedness versus rigid orthodoxy, one interpretation of Hahnemann versus another. Homoeopaths are fond of asserting that 'homoeopathy works', and no doubt many satisfied patients would wholeheartedly concur, but how can one demonstrate that it works better than other treatments, or compare one form of homoeopathic treatment with another? And what counts as 'working'? In the course of the debate (as can be seen from some of the extracts quoted here) there was reference to patients being 'cured', being 'satisfied', 'getting better', 'having a better quality of life'. Do these all mean the same thing? If not, what different levels or dimensions of improvement of the patient's state of health do they refer to?

Furthermore, it is as important for the growth of homoeopathic knowledge to be able to show what does not work as it is to show what works. In any case, there is no means by which homoeopaths can be sure about which approaches do not work. Homoeopathy is a not a therapy for those who are impatient for quick results, and it is impossible for the individual homoeopath to know what happens to the patient who simply does not complete the course of treatments thought necessary by the practitioner. (Did they not come back because they felt better already – or because they did not feel better and did not want to spend more time and money on something they regarded as useless?). Only the very confident and successful givers of seminars and master classes will publicise their known failures, so it is not surprising that newly qualified NMQ homoeopaths have sometimes complained of feeling isolated and disempowered. Probably this is true of new practitioners in medicine and other therapies as well, but the homoeopath has no clear means of knowing what sort of success rate he or she ought to be getting from any particular approach.

It would be insulting to a lively and self-critical professional group to suggest that they are not aware of this problem themselves. The issue of what kind of research strategy homoeopaths should use in order to advance and substantiate their body of professional knowledge has been under discussion for some time among members of the Society of Homoeopaths. Within the Society there appears to be little enthusiasm for the extension of biomedical research methodologies into homoeopathy in the expectation that this will increase practitioners' legitimacy in the eyes of the medical profession. David St George, for example, argues that randomised controlled trials are not appropriate for homoeopathy and that in any case NMQ homoeopaths should not be doing research solely as a defensive attempt to convince the medical profession. Research should be 'pragmatic real-world research' with the purpose of self-criticism and self-development, of continually improving the day-to-day practice of the profession (St George, 1994). Similarly, Bob Fordham has called for 'reflective practice', a concept developed in some other professions, such as nursing, which might, as he puts it, help homoeopathy to develop a professional culture that is 'comfortable with [this] tension between doubt and certainty' (Fordham, 1995, p. 343). It is certainly not the case that NMQ homoeopaths are unaware of the need to develop a research culture that will produce data to assist in the evaluation of different kinds of homoeopathic intervention.

Many debates take place within a particular professional or intellectual community which arouse enormous rancour at the time, yet are never resolved, merely fading into insignificance as some quite different issue becomes controversial (was the disagreement between F.R. Leavis and C.P. Snow about the 'two cultures' ever actually resolved?). I am not suggesting that 'reasonable consensus' about criteria for assessing outcomes of treatment would have settled the issue of 'classical' versus 'not just classical' approaches to prescribing once and for all. The process of debate in medical science tells us that this is seldom the case even for professions with well developed methods of assessment. The existence of broadly accepted methods of measuring medical outcome over time does not preclude vigorous debate about, say, the value of hormone replacement therapy (HRT), infant immunisation or other biomedical procedures. The point is not that such methodologies do away with indeterminacy (though they may reduce it) but that they allow people outside the professional group to understand the grounds of the debate and even to participate in it (as has certainly been the case with HRT and infant immunisation). What could the interested sympathiser (say, a patient who wanted to know which homoeopath to consult) make of the terms in which the debate about 'not just classical' prescribing was conducted? It is not a matter of finding the means to resolve an issue once and for all, but rather of finding the means by which the grounds of disagreement can be made plain even to those who are not practitioners themselves yet have a legitimate interest in the evaluation of procedures.

How was homoeopathy able to survive so long without any recognised and standardised modes of evaluating its procedures? The answer to this question is: in the same way that many other practical traditions of healing survived until very recently (including medicine itself). The demand for standardised principles of evaluation is a relatively modern one. Formerly, homoeopathic knowledge, as developed by NMQ homoeopaths, was (like many other forms of healing knowledge) advanced by charismatic practitioners who developed new remedies or ideas about prescribing. Different schools of thought developed as their pupils and associates followed this or that mode of practice. So long as the balance between fission and fusion remained fairly stable, the identity of homoeopathy as a healing therapy survived. Moreover until the founder members of the Society began to set up training schools in the 1970s, modes of homoeopathic education among NMQ homoeopaths in Britain were largely informal, more like apprenticeship, and in general the pressures for standardisation or conformity within this professional community were weak.

But recognition as a legitimate and respected profession, let alone state registration, now requires the development of standardised qualifications with formal methods of training and examination, which in turn requires some degree of agreement on core curricula and the nature of the homoeopathic knowledge base. With greater public emphasis on the accountability of professions, there are external pressures to develop demonstrable procedures for evaluating therapeutic interventions, in addition to pressures generated by the need to resolve internal debate.

The energies of the Research Committee of the Society of Homoeopaths have recently been directed to the issue of audit, and the Committee has been preparing to undertake a major audit of members' activities. Audit, as a form of inquiry, answers questions about the extent to which interventions have or have not achieved their intended aims. A form of audit that would both satisfy the external public need for accountability and contribute to fulfilling the internal professional need for the resolution of disagreement would depend on homoeopaths as a group managing to decide on common practical criteria for 'successful treatment'. As we have seen from some of the contributions to the debate, is an issue that is not totally clear at the moment, but consensus on this point might be easier to achieve than on the contentious issue of prescribing.

If the Research Committee is able to develop the audit process and achieve a good response rate from members, this may provide the kind of empirical data which might help break the deadlock in debates such as the one I have described. Audit will not satisfy the truly curious scientific mind, which will want to know why a treatment works, not just the extent to which it works. But it can throw light on the outcomes of different kinds of treatment – and light is a more useful form of energy than heat where intra-professional debates about practice are concerned. As one contributor to the debate about prescribing wrote: 'Don't criticise, audit!' (Meredith, 1992, p. 28.)

ACKNOWLEDGEMENTS

The investigation that provided much of the data for this paper took place as part of a wider study of professionalisation in complementary medicine carried out by Sarah Cant and myself. This project was funded by the Economic and Social Research Council, whose support I gratefully acknowledge. I would also like to acknowledge the cooperation of the Society of Homoeopaths, especially the kind help of their administrator, Mary Clarke.

REFERENCES

Bianchini, R. (1994) *The Homoeopath*, (53).
Brinkley, J. (1992) Letter. *Society of Homoeopaths Newsletter*, (June).
Chatfield, I. (1992) Letter. *Society of Homoeopaths Newsletter*, (March).
Crockett, P. (1992) Letter. *Society of Homoeopaths Newsletter*, (June).
Curtin, D., Lewith, G., Trenherz, F. and Burger, J. (1993) The great debate. *The Homoeopath*, **13**(1), 12–22
Fordham, B. (1995) The challenge of reflective practice. *The Homoeopath*, (56).
Harper, S. (1992) Letter. *Society of Homoeopaths Newsletter*, (June).
Logan, R. (1992) Letter. *Society of Homoeopaths Newsletter*, (December).

Meredith, F. (1992) Letter. *Society of Homoeopaths Newsletter*, (June).

Miles, M. (1992) Interviewed by M. Dean. *Society of Homoeopaths Newsletter*, (December).

Norland, M. (1992) Letter. *Society of Homoeopaths Newsletter*, (March).

Society of Homoeopaths (1991) Annual Report. Society of Homoeopaths, Northampton.

Southam, T. (1992) Letter. *Society of Homoeopaths Newsletter*, (March).

St George, D. (1994) Towards a research and development strategy for complementary medicine. *The Homoeopath*, (54), pp. 254–6.

<table>
<tr><td>13</td><td># Misconceptions about research in complementary medicine</td></tr>
</table>

13	# Misconceptions about research in complementary medicine

George Lewith

INTRODUCTION

Complementary therapists have often suggested that their 'whole person' approach to the treatment of illness cannot be evaluated using conventional clinical trials. In other words, alternative medicine requires alternative research. I will argue that, despite the claims of some practitioners, conventional research in complementary medicine is not only feasible, but necessary in order to answer questions of clinical importance. Moreover, I will make the case that research will be of benefit for promoting dialogue between complementary and conventional medicine. This dialogue has often been a sterile one: in the face of uncritical claims made by complementary practitioners about the benefits of their techniques, conventional doctors have sometimes retreated to a similarly uncritical stance that complementary medicine offers nothing of real value to patients and that it should not be practised or should even be outlawed (National Council Against Health Fraud, 1991). It is my belief that research can provide a common ground between these two extremes.

EVIDENCE, CRITICAL THINKING AND THE NATURE OF THE THERAPEUTIC RELATIONSHIP

It is apparent that a substantial proportion of clinicians – complementary and conventional alike – do not base their practice sufficiently on the best possible evidence. Though there are a number of reasons why opinion and personal experience are so widely favoured over rigorous research, one of the most interesting concerns the nature of the therapeutic relationship.

A patient, feeling unwell and vulnerable, seeks the advice of a clinician. This immediately places the clinician in a position of power and reinforces the idea that he or she has specialist knowledge. During the consultation, the greater the clinician's confidence, the greater the patient's belief and, therefore, the greater the placebo effect (Thomas, 1987; Beecher, 1955, 1961). The greater the placebo effect, the greater the chance of improvement. Consequently, the clinician's own belief is vindicated by the patient's apparent clinical response. This mitigates powerfully against a critical approach: doctors may even ignore good research if it contradicts the apparent 'truth' that confronts them in everyday clinical medicine. It might even be argued that clinicians must necessarily be uncritical. If they become too critical, and begin to lose their faith in their practice, they could lose some of their therapeutic power.

The problem is that the passionate, involved attitude that can be of such benefit in actually helping patients to get better can sometimes hinder reflection, critical thinking, and debate.

HOW MUCH DO COMPLEMENTARY PRACTITIONERS KNOW ABOUT RESEARCH?

Complementary practitioners may have strong opinions on research. They often make statements such as 'You can't do research on yoga'. Yet many qualified complementary practitioners have had little or no real training in science, clinical research or critical appraisal. Consequently their attitudes and approaches to research can be confused and biased.

There is a number of features of 'science' which is said to prevent conventional research in complementary medicine.

Scientific research has to be double-blind

Dossey (1995) provides an interesting example of this misconception when he refers to conventional medical research as 'double-blinding' and describes researchers as 'double-blinders.' This is clearly misleading, as most forms of research – surveys, laboratory experiments, epidemiological studies – are not and can not be done double-blind. One of the few types of research that can be undertaken on a double-blind basis is the randomised controlled trial (RCT). But RCTs do not have to be conducted blindly and, in many cases, it would not be possible to do so: who, after all, would want a blind surgeon? Yet, practitioners and commentators in both conventional and complementary medicine repeatedly state that RCTs have to be double-blind. This is most obvious when terms are used interchangeably: 'there is increasing pressure on alternative therapy to document effects by using the randomized double-blind controlled clinical trial, in the following just called the "controlled clinical trial" ' (Lausø, 1994).

Scientific research requires placebo controls

Thinking about placebo controls for many complementary therapies – massage would be a good example – strains creativity, credibility and medical ethics. Thus a perceived need for placebo controls is a major disincentive to research for many complementary practitioners. Lazarides (1995) suggests that unless research is placebo controlled ('follows the rules' of the 'randomised double-blind placebo controlled trial') it is unlikely that it will be 'embraced by mainstream medicine.' Again, this would only be true of RCT research on efficacy and, again, only a proportion of RCTs involve control groups that receive a placebo or other mimic therapy. As a simple example, one RCT published in a conventional journal examined the value of respiratory rehabilitation for patients with severe but stable chronic obstructive pulmonary disease (Goldstein et al., 1994). The treatment group were rehabilitated as inpatients for 8 weeks and supervised as outpatients for 16 weeks. The control group received standard care. There was no attempt to use a placebo.

Scientific research must involve standardised treatment

Complementary practitioners generally vary their treatment from patient to patient, even when patients have the same conventional diagnosis. If treatments in research have to be standardised, and in some way that seems artificial, this obviously presents a very serious challenge to research in complementary medicine. Launsø (1994) states that 'treatment [in RCTs] must be reduced to isolated and measurable techniques' and that the 'method of assessment determines [a priori] which treatments are regarded as acceptable'. Similarly, Lazarides (1995) claims that 'standard clinical trial methodology . . . requires a single treatment formula for all patients with a particular Western diagnosis'. But neither author gives any reasons why the treatment used in an RCT has to be standardised and measurable. There are numerous counter-examples. For instance, Tyrer and colleagues compared two models of mental health care provision: close supervision by nominated key workers and standard follow-up from psychiatric and social services (Tyrer et al., 1995). The health professionals involved treated the patients as they would normally – on a case-by-case basis responding to individual needs. They did not therefore use an 'isolated and measurable technique' or a 'single treatment formula.'

Scientific research is about objective measurement

It has been suggested that research can only involve objective outcome measures – blood pressure and heart rate, for example – rather than quality of life or feelings of relaxation. Dossey (1995) states, 'Science is about facts, not feelings.' Mercer, Long and Smith (1995) suggest that 'the use of medically defined "objective" outcome measures avoids any reliance on subjective patient reports of their condition'. This is untrue: many RCTs rely exclusively on patient report. An example might be Foster *et al.*, (1994), who studied the effect of a special type of dressing on diabetic neuropathy. Outcome was assessed in terms of pain and quality of life. No attempt was made to find any objective changes resulting from the use of the dressings. Similarly, many other forms of research – qualitative research is an obvious example – involve asking questions about subjective states.

Research involves reductionism whereby the world becomes a mechanical machine

Complementary practitioners think of their techniques as holistic and based upon a 'systems theory' approach. Some methodologists sympathetic to complementary medicine have claimed that research inevitably involves a model contrary to this view. This point is perhaps made most forcefully by Heron (1986) who talks of a 'linear univariate causal view – this single variable causing changes in this or that single variable – [which] gives a unidimensional and hence a limited and misleading view of . . . multidimensional reality. To see the world as a self-contained mechanical realm compounded of sets of point-to-point linear cause–effect sequences is out of date in theoretical physics . . . it is odd that it should still have any claim in the scientific basic of therapeutics'. Similarly, Mercer, Long and Smith (1995) claim that the RCT 'fits with the theoretical assumptions contained in the biomedical model [such as] the reduction of the body to its constituent parts'. On examination, it is not at all clear that scientific research does presuppose a tightly defined set of assumptions about the body or reality in general. Some research programmes, such as the human genome project, do appear to be reductionist; others, such as research on perception in clinical psychology, do not. If it is true that even the RCT is predicated on mechanical, linear, point-to-point causal relationships, or the reduction of the body to its constituent parts, it would become difficult to explain the existence of RCTs on psychotherapy (Winston *et al.*, 1994) and prayer (Byrd, 1988): the former consists of an interactive dialogue between practitioner and patient and is therefore indisputably non-linear; the latter can hardly be said to presuppose either mechanistic Newtonian causality or the reduction of the whole to its parts.

THE DIALOGUE

One of the main problems that occurs in attempting to overcome the differences between clinical research science and complementary medicine is that of language and education. All too often complementary medical practitioners feel that their ignorance about clinical research methodology presents an insurmountable problem should they attempt to design a clinical trial. Clinical research scientists tend to look upon complementary practitioners' attitudes to research as entirely inappropriate.

However, complementary practitioners are justified in having some grounds for concern. Well-known incidents such as the Bristol Cancer Help Centre study, where, arguably, researchers subverted the scientific process in order to denigrate complementary medicine (Bagenal *et al.*, 1990), show that research can be a political as well as scientific undertaking. Often, however, problems in complementary medicine research are more subtle. My first experience of this was an attempt to design a clinical trial on acupuncture and irritable bowel syndrome. I wanted to use a traditional Chinese approach using as many points as I needed, but the physician with whom I was working wished to circumscribe the number of points I could use. In consequence I would have been testing a very limited form of acupuncture.

I have argued consistently over the last 14 years that if one is going to test complementary medicine in the context of clinical trials, then the best available therapy should be tested rather than some conventional physician's view of what that therapy might or might not be (Lewith and Machin, 1983). This pragmatic approach to complementary medicine has resulted in some great successes: for instance, the study by Meade and colleagues (1990) which analysed the effect of chiropractic in the management of low back pain. Complementary practitioners are quite correct in assuming that some conventional physicians marginalise complementary therapeutic interventions by simply failing to understand its entirety and complexity. Nevertheless, in spite of the many limitations of clinical research, it is quite clear that competent, pragmatic studies can be effected. These studies take our understanding of complementary medicine further forward by demonstrating its clinical relevance. They can also provide 'common ground' in the debate and dialogue between complementary and conventional medicine.

CONCLUSION

A divide has existed between complementary practitioners and conventional doctors in their attitudes to research (this now appears slowly, to be being bridged). Both have historically adopted entrenched views, neither of which can be realistically sustained. It is my belief that the particular and unusual circumstances surrounding the consultation make for great difficulties when attempting to adopt a self-critical and evidence-led approach to therapeutic interventions.

If the belief exhibited by many complementary practitioners has an important therapeutic role, the attitude encultured by clinical researchers may result in a more negative therapeutic encounter, and consequently a diminution in the practitioner's benefit to the patient. As such, introducing a research culture into complementary medicine may have real drawbacks for patients. In spite of this potential problem, complementary practitioners must look at their therapies with an eye to positive and critical evaluation. Through dialogue, both within and between the professions, we will begin to develop a more rational approach to therapeutic decisions. This approach needs to give us the strength and confidence to reject dogma if it is shown to be unsustainable, without devaluing the humanity and compassion that underpin all good medical practice.

REFERENCES

Bagenal, E.S., Easton, D.F., Harris, E. *et al.* (1990) Survival of patients with breast cancer attending the Bristol Cancer Help Centre. *Lancet*, **336**, 606–10.

Beecher, H.K. (1955) The powerful placebo. *Journal of the American Medical Association*, **159**, 1602–6.

Beecher, H.K. (1961) Surgery as placebo. *Journal of the American Medical Association*, **176**, 1102–7.

Byrd, R. (1988) Positive therapeutic effects of intercessory prayer in a coronary care unit population. *Southern Medical Journal*, **91**, 826–9.

Dossey, L. (1995) How should alternative therapies be evaluated? *Alternative Therapies in Health and Medicine*, **1**, 6–10.

Foster, A.V., Eaton, C., McConville, D.O. and Edmonds, M.E. (1994) Application of OpSite film: a new and effective treatment of painful diabetic neuropathy. *Diabetic Medicine*, **11**, 768–72.

Goldstein, R.S., Gort, E.H., Stubbing, D. *et al.* (1994) Randomised controlled trial of respiratory rehabilitation. *Lancet*, **344**, 1394–7.

Heron, J. (1986) Critique of conventional research methodology. *Complementary Medical Research*, **1**, 12–22.

Launsø, L. (1994) How to kiss a monster, in *Studies in Alternative Therapy 1* (eds H. Johannessen *et al.*), Odense University Press, Odense, Denmark.

Lazarides, L. (1995) Position paper: nutritional therapy research. Society for the Promotion of Nutritional Therapy, Heathfield, UK.

Lewith, G.T. and Machin, D. (1983) On the evaluation of the clinical effects of acupuncture. *Pain*, **16**, 111–27.

Meade, D.W., Dyer, S., Brown, N.E.W. *et al.* (1990) Low back pain of mechanical origin: randomised comparison of chiropractic and hospital outpatient treatment. *British Medical Journal*, **300**, 1431–7.

Mercer, G., Long, A.F. and Smith, I.J. (1995) *Researching and evaluating complementary therapies: the state of the debate.* Nuffield Institute for Health, Leeds.

National Council Against Health Fraud (1991) Acupuncture. The position paper of the National Council Against Health Fraud. *Clinical Journal of Pain*, **7**, 162–6.

Thomas, K.B. (1987) General practice consultations: is there any point in being positive? *British Medical Journal*, **294**, 1200–2.

Tyrer, P., Morgan, J., Van Horn, E. *et al.* (1995) A randomised controlled study of close monitoring of vulnerable psychiatric patients. *Lancet*, **345**, 756–9.

Winston, A., Laikin, M., Pollack, J. *et al.* (1994) Short-term psychotherapy of personality disorders. *American Journal of Psychiatry*, **151**, 190–4.

Science and critical discourse in chiropractic: a short history

14

Maria Hondras

Skepticemia – an uncommon generalized disorder of low infectivity. Medical school education is likely to confer life-long immunity.

Petr Skrabanek and James McCormick (1989)

INTRODUCTION

For more than a century, chiropractors have wrestled with the concepts of philosophy and science. The founder of chiropractic, D.D. Palmer, characterised his offering as 'science, art, and philosophy,' (Keating, 1992; Palmer, 1910), and his son, the 'Developer' (B.J. Palmer) preached a philosophy of 'pure, straight and unadulterated chiropractic,' which bound the doctor of chiropractic (DC) to spiritualism and dogmatic clinical theories (Keating, 1992). Many leaders of chiropractic's educational reform and accreditation movement (1973–1974) offered a philosophy that emphasised the value of basic scientific knowledge, but rejected clinical research as irrelevant, impractical and too expensive for the poverty-stricken chiropractic colleges (Budden, 1948; Homewood, 1979; 1988; Keating, 1992). Others (Hildebrandt, 1967; Janse, 1976; Shrader, 1968; Watkins, 1944) held that clinical research and experimentation ought to provide a knowledge base for clinical decision making, and that the responsibility for conducting clinical research rested with chiropractors (Keating, 1992).

Many argue that all health care disciplines must embrace the notion of providing evidence for decisions. The information explosion allows lifelong learning habits for all people. In this paper I examine the critical discourse that links the professionalisation and education of chiropractors with science in chiropractic. I hope to underline the intensity of the warning sounded by Ebrall (1995) that, as the third largest health care provider group in the United States, the profession's future is far from being assured, and that chiropractors should be deeply concerned with the challenges of change the profession is facing. The intraprofessional discord over 'super-straights,' 'straights,' and 'mixers' will not be discussed, although it is important to remember that there is a large faction in the profession that treats only the subluxation, denounces the diagnostic process and makes no claims of treating illness. Rather, they are in the business of 'subluxation removal'. Nor will this paper review the professional identity crisis that has emerged of late, between 'primary care providers', 'neuromusculoskeletal specialists', and 'any other specialists' within chiropractic. Chiropractors have a long history of circling the wagons, and then turning in – to fire. Perhaps governments, managed care organisations and, ultimately, the public will sort out who chiropractors are, and what they treat, before chiropractors do. I believe that our scope of practice will be sharply defined by outside forces and that the chiropractic colleges that survive the next quarter of a century will be remarkably different from what they are today. I also believe that if sufficient attention is not paid to the socialisation of chiropractors to scientific principles, chiropractic will not survive for a second hundred years.

LESSONS FROM THE FIRST HUNDRED YEARS

As the twentieth century dawned, health care in the midwestern United States included a wide assortment of theories, methods and practitioners (Keating, 1995a). A variety of health care practitioners were available, such as 'regular,' orthodox or 'allopathic' practitioners; physicians and surgeons; eclectic medical practitioners; homeopathic physicians; osteopaths; magnetic healers; nature cure practitioners; Christian Scientists and faith healers; and patent medicine vendors. The Flexner Report, which would describe the deplorable state of medical education in the USA, was still ten years in the future. Although the growing European traditions of laboratory science, sanitation and conservatism had begun to influence the content and quality of several university-based colleges of medicine along the eastern seaboard of the USA, those influences had not reached most practitioners along the Mississippi River (Keating, 1995a). As Keating describes:

> The gentler European alternatives to America's heroic medical methods were the province of the 'irregulars'. In many states, medical licensing laws, which had been repealed by public demand in the first 30 years of the nineteenth century, were reappearing, but were not yet so widely enforced that they prevented most irregulars from practicing their crafts at the turn of the century.

As the nineteenth century drew to a close, with few exceptions (e.g. the National School of Chiropractic and the Cook Country Hospital in Chicago), chiropractors were denied access to the institutions that might have permitted greater socialisation to the attitudes and demeanour of the emerging science of medicine (Keating, 1995b). By 1905, just ten years after the birth of the chiropractic profession, a number of students at the Palmer School became disenchanted with B.J. Palmer's administration of the school, particularly the religious fervour that pervaded the nine-month curriculum and the lack of science to support the chiropractic art. In 1906, John F. Howard founded the National School of Chiropractic and began the tradition of 'rational chiropractic.' Along with William Charles Schulze, and Arthur L. Forster, Howard and his newly formed faculty introduced physiological therapeutics into the chiropractic curriculum, including procedures involving light, heat, cold, electricity, water, nutritional interventions, and exercise regimens. The school was renamed the National College of Chiropractic in 1920 and became a strong proponent for improvement in the educational process, emphasising basic science instruction (Keating, 1995a).

Despite the efforts of Howard, Schulze and Forster, organised medicine-enacted basic science legislation that threatened the viability of the chiropractic profession, as well as osteopathy and naturopathy. It was not until 1935, at the National Chiropractic Association's (NCA) Fortieth Anniversary Convention, that a 'classic reformation' was launched (Gibbons, 1985; Keating, 1993). From this meeting evolved the NCA's Committee on Educational Standards, forerunner of today's Council on Chiropractic Education (CCE). Although educational reform has carried the profession from 1935 to the end of the twentieth century, the reshaping of chiropractic education and the professionalisation process continue today.

Legitimate, sustained, scientific research in chiropractic is a rather recent phenomenon (Dishman, 1985; Keating, 1992; Keating, 1995b). However, throughout chiropractic's 100 year history, the terms 'research' and 'science' have been among the most popular in the literature of chiropractic and have often been used in ways that are unfamiliar to most scientists (Keating, 1995b). There are numerous examples of proclamations, journals, newsletters, textbooks and public relations copy that include scientific verbiage but have little to do with the actual conduct and reporting of research or with critical thinking about scholarly, scientific or technological advances. Precious few were other than self-proclaimed, uncritically published or unpublished, uncontrolled observations of manipulative therapy (Keating, 1995b). Furthermore, this illegitimate science was widely disseminated among practitioners, and in the hands of chiropractic marketeers this 'evidence' took on a life of its own (Keating, 1995b).

One report was published in the booklet entitled *Chiropractic Statistics*, and distributed by an advertising firm that handled the promotional campaigns of the American Society of Chiropractors in the early 1930s. The booklet presented descriptive outcome data for dozens of acute and chronic conditions treated by chiropractors, from 'ACNE' to 'UREMIA' (Anon. 1925; Keating, 1995b). These data were reprinted in a 1929 pamphlet distributed throughout the profession, *Health Through Chiropractic* (American Society of Chiropractors, 1929), and were touted as scientific evidence of the validity and effectiveness of chiropractic theory and practice 11 years after their original appearance in *Chiropractic Statistics*. Furthermore, they were reprinted again in a 1938 hardbound book of testimonials (Keating, 1995b). The summary overview states:

> This report covers 99,976 cases reported by 412 chiropractors in 110 specific conditions. These cases resulted as follows:
>
> 84,571 or 84.59% Recovered or greatly improved.
> 14,554 or 14.56% Condition unchanged.
> 851 or 00.85% Died.

The death rate, equivalent to 8.5 per 1000 compares with a general death rate of 12.3 per 1000 throughout the United States for the year of 1923, the last year for which final figures are available. Deducting 1.15 – the death rate from accident, homicide and suicide – the national disease rate was 11.15 per 1000 under all forms of treatment and 8.5 under chiropractic, the latter rate being 23.7% lower (Anon. 1925).

Methodological considerations – such as the criteria used in arriving at the various diagnoses, types of chiropractic intervention, concurrent care, and criteria for judging recovery – were not reported; in short, it would have been impossible for anyone to attempt to replicate these findings (Keating, 1995b). The meaningfulness of the survey information was never challenged by chiropractors. As Keating (1995b) asserts

> Most practitioners of the adjustive arts had little exposure to the scientific community and no opportunity to form more sophisticated attitudes about the scientific method. If chiropractors in the first half of this century considered that clinical research was important at all, the examples provided from within the profession did little to expand their awareness of scientific methodology, and did much to reinforce their uncritical, *a priori* beliefs in the validity of chiropractic theory.

Unfortunately, as the second half of this century comes to a close, many chiropractic students and practitioners have no compulsion about utilising as evidence the results of reports such as *Chiropractic Statistics*, particularly because of 'the large sample size'.

PROPONENTS OF RESEARCH IN CHIROPRACTIC

Fifty years after the birth of the chiropractic profession, C.O. Watkins (1946) published a critical treatise exposing the lack of a commitment to the scholarly pursuits of science, and the threat this posed for unity in the profession. His comparison of the scientific and philosophical movements has not outlived its usefulness 50 years later (Table 14.1).

Having participated in the early reform efforts of the NCA (1934–1944), Watkins came to appreciate that a commitment to scholarship was missing from chiropractic's social and political structures. While recognising that professional associations had many demanding and complex functions and purposes, he countered that none was more fundamental nor more patient-oriented than the development of the knowledge base by which clinicians practise (Keating, 1992). In his self-published discourse, *The Basic Principles of Chiropractic Government*, (1944) Watkins explains his views on the fundamental role and responsibility of chiropractic professional organisations to take charge of scientific development (Keating, 1992). This responsibility, he suggests, derives from the obligation of every member of the profession to advance the knowledge base in chiropractic. Moreover, he notes, the demands of clinical research are such that only with an adequate organisation of the profession can significant progress be expected (Keating, 1992).

During the 1960s and 1970s, many people repeatedly called for the chiropractic colleges to assume a larger role in consolidating the knowledge and power base of the profession, especially in the areas of research and professional standards (DeBoer, 1983). By 1978, the *Journal of Manipulative and Physiological Therapeutics (JMPT)* became the first, and to this day the only, chiropractic journal indexed by *Index Medicus*. The first editor of the *JMPT* repeatedly challenged chiropractors to become actively and progressively engaged in applying the methods of scientific inquiry in furthering chiropractic's claims to knowledge and in improving techniques (Hildebrandt, 1982). Although manipulation was recognised as enjoying an extremely strong empirical track record (Hildebrandt, 1978), there were little data to evaluate this clinical approach to health and to the treatment of disease (Hildebrandt, 1979). Although the *JMPT* would be the scholarly choice to disseminate such information, the circulation of this journal has never reached more than 10% of the chiropractic profession. Indeed, this is probably an overestimate, as there are only 4000 paid subscribers at the time of this writing, many of whom are not chiropractors (Lawrence, personal communication).

It was almost 40 years after Watkins published his 'natural characteristics of scientific and philosophical movements' that a critical discourse re-emerged on the dearth of evidence and the need for a research infrastructure to support the education and professionalisation of chiropractors. In 1983, DeBoer challenged the adequacy of the profession's leadership (DeBoer, 1983). He invited college leaders to revisit three categories of collegiate problems: (1) clinical training, (2) research and (3) faculty, curriculum, students and administration. DeBoer advocated rearranging clinical training to revolve around a select group of 'clinical professors' and that this would help solve many of the problems besetting clinical training and research at the colleges. He reminded

Table 14.1 Natural characteristics of scientific and philosophical movements[a]

Scientific movement	Philosophical movement
Fundamental Basis	
Has as its basis the fundamental principles, attitudes and methods of science.	Has as its basis a teaching doctrine, dogma or creed. Disregards the principles, attitudes and methodology of science.
Ultimate objective	
Endeavours to establish itself as an accepted branch of science.	Endeavours to establish itself as a separate and distinct movement of science.
Attitude towards education	
In science, education is paramount. The success of the scientific movement is dependent upon its membership's knowledge and will to search for new knowledge. Education is a continuous endeavour to the scientist.	Unimportant. Once students are thoroughly indoctrinated with the basic doctrine and methods, their education is complete. They then become evangelists to indoctrinate others.
Attitude towards research	
The search for new knowledge and better methods is the strongest motivating force in science. The search is broad in scope, and new facts are sought and evaluated wherever found in the field of science. Useful knowledge and methods are incorporated into one's scientific endeavours. Accepts only facts that have been demonstrated by scientific methods.	Cares little for research since one's concept or methods are not going to develop. If any research is done, it is only for the purpose of proving what one already believes. It is always within the scope of the basic doctrine. One regards as fact anything that is contained in the original doctrine.
Public approach	
Publishes and explains demonstrated facts. (Cinema, press or radio may then dramatise them.) Does not advertise in the trade sense of the word or evangelise in the religious sense of the word. Aggressive within the movement: humble towards the public. Makes no claim.	Publishes, evangelises and often advertises its creed, doctrine or dogma in an effort to convert the public to its concept. Ignores or belittles demonstrated facts if in conflict with its doctrine. Aggressive towards the public. Claims everything contained in its doctrine.
Cohesiveness of movement	
Membership drawn closer together to exchange knowledge. May divide to form new branches covering specialised endeavours, but always maintaining close liaison with the main body.	Membership tends to break up into cults around new teachings or doctrines. Once separated, these never reunite on basic differences. May cooperate on matters in which the doctrines do not conflict.

[a]Reprinted from Watkins (1946).

us that training a cadre of clinicians in the scientific method is a slow and demanding process, and pointed to the timetable deemed reasonable in 1979 by the World Health Organisation:

A scientific institution with some capability for research can be set up in about 5 years. Scientific workers with some research experience can be trained in about 10 years. It takes a generation or so of educational and cultural change to foster the personal qualities needed to solve practical problems by scientific methods.

DeBoer, (1983)

Ironically, the major force behind the research effort from the colleges has been the separation of researchers from the rest of the faculty. Chiropractic colleges are the only health care professional schools that I know of that have separate and distinct 'research departments'. Perhaps our chiropractic leaders did not heed the advice of DeBoer because he is not a chiropractor. Or perhaps the medium through which DeBoer chose to publish his 'notes from the (chiropractic college's) underground' – the *JMPT* – did not attain sufficient readership. If students, practitioners and leaders in the chiropractic profession missed this voice crying in the wilderness, they have no excuse to have missed the message from the prolific discourse offered during 'the Keating years'.

Like DeBoer, Joseph C. Keating, Jr holds a PhD rather than a DC degree. However, for the past ten years, Keating has flooded the chiropractic literature in a sufficient variety of chiropractic journals, magazines and newsletters that we can no longer deny having heard his arguments. Keating has published widely about the traditional barriers to research in chiropractic and the need to develop a cadre of practitioner-scientists (Keating, 1987b; 1988; 1989a, b, c; 1990). Keating and others have repeatedly identified the steps necessary to sustain the research effort of the colleges (Keating, 1987a; 1989 a, b, c, d, e, f; Keating *et al.*, 1986). The need for qualified research personnel tops the list. Moreover, a competitive salary structure must be implemented to support not only investigators, but also support personnel. Additional funds need to be mobilised for consultants, seminars, workshops and symposia. Collaborative relationships between basic scientists and clinicians, as well as between investigators in different colleges must be formed. Investigators from chiropractic institutions must maintain visibility within their respective disciplines by participating in international symposia and contributing to the literature. All of these things are part of the baggage one inherits when one buys into a substantive research effort (DeBoer, 1983).

By 1988, Keating was challenging the ethos of the profession, this time in his address to the House of Delegates of the American Chiropractic Association, reprinted in the *American Journal of Chiropractic Medicine (AJCM)*. Keating decried that the single, most self-defeating concept in this profession is epitomised by the phrase 'chiropractic works.' (Keating, 1989f). He argued that this attitude, which says that 'we already know it works', does more to inhibit progress in the science, art and philosophy of chiropractic and does more to tarnish the public image of the chiropractor than any other current obstacle (Keating, 1989f). Some of the reasons for Keating's proclamation bear repeating:

> Imagine that we stopped claiming that 'chiropractic works.' Imagine that our students and faculty and practitioners made no specific claims for chiropractic care except those which were strongly supported by clinical research data. I believe that we have good reason to anticipate that some of our research data would exceed our current expectations, that some of our methods would not be as useful as we have supposed, and that others should be discontinued as harmful. But if we had ceased to make unsupported claims, we would be motivated as never before to carefully, critically, objectively explore the marvellous potential of the chiropractic science and art. Our future researchers should not start out by assuming that we already know where our research will take us, nor what it will tell us. We must be ready for discovery, for the unexpected, for the possibilities of new theories and new methods which we cannot yet even imagine. This is part of the wonder of our clinical science: its mystery and its uncertainty.

> Imagine that chiropractic students were not repeatedly instructed that 'chiropractic works.' Suppose we encouraged them to explore what does and doesn't work in chiropractic? Yet today, all too few students or doctors develop the motivation, the attitude, and the skills necessary to read and/or conduct serious clinical research. Why should they? They already 'know it works.' Why would anyone invest the time and the effort and the money to develop expertise in clinical research if he or she was already convinced of the outcome of that research? How can we expect to motivate and inspire the next generation towards careers in the applied science of chiropractic if we insist that we already know what the results of our research will be? Why should the field doctor stay current with chiropractic scientific literature if he or she already knows that 'it works?' We must not permit the belief that 'chiropractic works' to undercut the motivation to systematically and objectively explore the chiropractic healing art.

> Keating (1989f)

In a similar vein, DeBoer (1988) offered harsh criticism of our institutional leaders in his commentary 'Eine kleine nacht musing', by proclaiming that chiropractic institutions are run today as they have always been run – as technical trade-training schools. 'To be sure, chiropractic colleges are, without doubt, the world's best trade schools. They are very high class operations, with well motivated students, highly educated faculty and a well-focused college-like atmosphere. They have not, however, made the transition into legitimate professional education, with serious scholarship, research, and service, which are the hallmarks of the traditional professional institutions.'

There have been small-scale responses to improve the fragile research infrastructure at chiropractic colleges. The Foundation for Chiropractic Education and Research (FCER) has made several contributions, despite the fact that few past or present members of its board of directors have held advanced training in education or research. From 1983 to 1995, FCER awarded fellowships for the pursuit of advanced degrees to more than 40 chiropractors. In 1990, FCER selected the Corporate Health Policies Group (CHPG) of Bethesda, Maryland, to conduct a study to evaluate Federal funding policies and programmes and their relationship to chiropractic, ostensibly because the perception was that US government agencies were discriminating against proposals from chiropractic institutions. The results of the CHPG report were that chiropractic has not developed the necessary scientific and academic infrastructure to support large-scale Federal grants for research and academic development (Corporate Health Policies Group, 1991).

Even though critical discussions of the importance of training clinician-scholars have been numerous for more than ten years, only a handful of chiropractors have been supported for advanced training in research in the USA and Canada, and even fewer outside North America. If the leaders of the profession have not heard of the barriers to a sustained research effort in chiropractic, nor of the proposed solutions to these barriers, it is not because they have not been identified. If chiropractic leaders believe that Federal funding will by itself sustain the research effort of the profession into the third millennium, they are mistaken.

BARRIERS TO PROFESSIONALISATION AT THE CLOSE OF THE TWENTIETH CENTURY

Historically, chiropractic institutions have been run by chiropractors. By 1996, most chiropractic colleges met the CCE accreditation standards for 'teaching research' with one two-credit or three-credit research course in the core curriculum. In many colleges, this is the sum and substance of the institution's commitment to research. Moreover, very few chiropractors – including DC faculty, clinicians and administrators, who graduated from professional training more than 6–8 years ago had taken even a token course in research methodology or evaluating the literature, let alone additional graduate training in education or research.

For allopathic physicians, the fundamental problem was identified by Gehlbach more than 15 years ago (1980):

Medical literature is widely acknowledged as a major source of information and continuing education for postgraduate physicians. They must 'keep current' with professional journals in order to remain abreast of the latest . . . in etiologic hunches, novel diagnostic procedures, and therapeutic trends. Yet for all the importance attached to reading the literature, there is little in medical school or postgraduate training that teaches physicians to interpret medical studies intelligently. Even the most diligent readers will be little better for their efforts if they lack the ability to sort the valuable contributions from trivial or misleading articles.

It is imperative that educators and practitioners of complementary therapies move beyond the 'medical', as Gehlbach describes, and include health science literature from all health care disciplines, that is, reports of original research. We must be willing to admit that we rarely interpret the methods and results sections of original research (if we read peer-reviewed, indexed journals at all), but rather skim the abstract, then skip directly to the conclusion and discussion sections. We must assimilate the information as completely understood: the aims, findings and meaning of the findings.

In a survey of Australian chiropractors, Jamison (1991) explored practitioners' perceptions of the ability of various research designs to act as a guide to the effectiveness and safety of clinical interventions. With one exception, the group with 11–20 years clinical experience who regarded case–control studies as providing the most useful information upon which to predict clinical efficacy, all respondent groups regarded previous personal experience as the most useful guide to ascertaining whether an intervention is likely to be clinically effective. None of the respondent groups regarded randomised clinical trials as the best source of information about efficacy, and cohort studies were regarded as the least efficient research design. In addition, previous personal experience and physiological logic were the evidence of choice to predict the probable safety of an intervention. Jamison concludes that the 20% response rate to this survey does not weaken her conclusion that chiropractors may not adequately appreciate the usefulness of scientifically acceptable data collection and analyses as information sources for clinical decision making (Jamison, 1991).

Although the profession has made great strides in many areas of education, research and patient care, it is incumbent upon educators and practitioners to learn the language utilised by health care professionals in the USA and throughout the world. When the opportunity arises to communicate with other health professionals about the benefits of chiropractic care, it is inappropriate to claim that 'the Manga report' or 'the Meade study' (conclusively) demonstrates that chiropractic is cost effective for low back conditions. We must not allow these misinterpretations of the efforts by Manga and colleagues (1993) and Meade and colleagues (1990). When we say 'research shows' or 'research proves' let us be clear about the research we have read. We must evaluate the strength of the evidence. Our patients and our students deserve no less. If we are going to communicate with our students, colleagues and patients about efficacy, efficiency, effectiveness, coordinated care, primary care, prevalence, incidence, cost-effectiveness, outcomes, quality of life, and risk–benefit decisions, we must not abuse the intended meaning of these concepts and this language. Perhaps most important, it is not sufficient to believe simply that 'it works, my patients get better'. What does 'it' mean, and how do we define 'works' or 'better'?

Given the dearth of formal training in the scientific method and the skills to critically evaluate reports in the open literature, and because chiropractic institutions have not aligned themselves with established health science centres, colleges and universities, it is unlikely that the profession will survive the scrutiny and accountability of the changing face of health care. For educators and practitioners of acupuncture, homeopathy and other complementary therapies, these barriers to critical thinking and evidence-based medicine are no less important.

We must possess the tools to evaluate the health science literature. We must think critically before we can teach our students critical thinking. It is a sad commentary that in 1996 the vast majority of chiropractors lack the sophistication to evaluate reports of original research.

CRITICAL DISCOURSE FOR THE NEW MILLENNIUM

All health care professional curricula are destined for change as we move into the third millennium. The challenge for the future is in mastering information: finding effective ways to gather, store, retrieve, evaluate, distil and select information in ways that enhance cognition and support action rather than increase confusion and indecision. Science and informatics will guide educational reform for health care professionals in the twenty-first century.

The call to health care professionals to improve their ability to interpret information related to their particular discipline has occurred over only the past three or four decades. We have one very small tier of scientist-educators at chiropractic institutions worldwide. Not only is the number of chiropractic researchers desperately small, there is little evidence that the next generation of chiropractic researchers will be sufficient not only to replace the currently active and ageing research fraternity but also to grow the discipline. The opportunities for mentorship are severely limited in some chiropractic colleges and non-existent in others.

It is difficult to assess the impact of the research effort from the colleges on clinical practice. Although the circulation of *JMPT* is low and although we in the research community most often end up 'talking to ourselves' at national and international scientific symposia, we would like to believe that results from original research are impacting upon clinical practice and the patients we serve. For example, a quick scan of the *JMPT* for the past two years reveals at least a dozen reports of original research related to diagnostic testing, including: the responsiveness and clinical/research applicability of the Revised Oswestry Disability Questionnaire and the Dallas Pain Questionnaire (Haas *et al.*, 1995); the reliability of lumbar mobility measures, utilising both high and low technology (Stude, Goertz and Gallinger, 1994; Breum, 1995); evaluation of the clinical utility of leg length inequality measure (DeWitt *et al.*, 1994; Rhodes, 1995b); reliability and accuracy of the tissue compliance meter (Kawchuk and Herzog, 1995); gait analysis of sacroiliac patients (Herzog and Conway, 1994); and reliability studies of digital videofluoroscopy (Thorkeldsen and Breen, 1994). In an ideal world, results from these studies would be systematically reviewed in light of the weight of evidence, and if the diagnostic test were found unreliable or invalid, with little or no clinical utility, then the logical conclusion would be to abandon the test. However, there are no data indicating that the results of research are incorporated into clinical practice.

In response to these challenges, we must embrace a commitment to scholarship at chiropractic institutions and we must explore new ways to disseminate information to practitioners. Strong consideration should be given to the strategies adopted at our sister schools in Canada, Western Europe and Australasia. We must consider aligning ourselves with established institutions of higher learning. The culture of science exists within the university system and this is the most effective channel to influence future generations of chiropractors. Within the university system we will be able to train future researchers and college administrators to sustain the educational reform needed for the twenty-first century.

> It is said that nature abhors a vacuum. On the level of psychology this can be translated to mean that the human mind abhors a vacuum of knowledge, and when we are confronted with a striking unknown, like Stonehenge or Callanish, we humans have a profound tendency to rush headlong in with explanations for which there is no significant evidence – even to the point of making up evidence to justify our explanations. Although it does not always succeed in doing so, true science is all about combating this tendency of ours. The scientific method is our best strategy against jumping to hasty conclusions. We scientists also love to rush in wherever there is great mystery, but we try to do so with great caution.

> M. Scott Peck (1995)

REFERENCES

American Society of Chiropractors (1929) *Health Through Chiropractic*, American Society of Chiropractors, Columbus, OH.

Anon. (1925) *Chiropractic Statistics*, Chiropractic Research & Review Service, Indianapolis.

Breum, J., Wiberg, J. and Bolton, J.E. (1995) Reliability and concurrent validity of the BROM II for measuring lumbar mobility. *Journal of Manipulative and Physiological Therapies*, **18**, 497–502.

Budden, W.A. (1948) Comment on a proposal. *Journal of the National Chiropractic Association*, **18**, 24.

Corporate Health Policies Group (1991) An evaluation of Federal funding policies and programs and their relationship to the chiropractic profession. Foundation for Chiropractic Education and Research, Arlington, VA.

DeBoer, K.F. (1983) Notes from the (chiropractic college's) underground. *Journal of Manipulative and Physiological Therapies*, **6**, 147–50.

DeBoer, K.F. (1988) Eine kleine Nacht musing. *American Journal of Chiropractic Medicine*, **1**, 41–3.

DeWitt, J.K., Osterbauer, P.J., Stelmach, G.E. and Fuhr, A.W. (1994) Optoelectric measurement of changes in leg length inequality resulting from isolation tests. *Journal of Manipulative and Physiological Therapies*, **17**, 530–8.

Dishman, R.W. (1985) Review of the literature supporting a scientific basis for the chiropractic subluxation complex. *Journal of Manipulative Physiological Therapies*, **8**, 163–74.

Ebrall, P. (1995) Chiropractic and second hundred years: a shiny new millennium or the return of the dark ages? *Journal of Manipulative Physiological Therapies*, **18**, 631–5.

Gehlbach, S.H. Teaching residents to read the medical literature. *Journal of Medical Education*, **55**, 362–5.

Gibbons, R.W. (1985) Chiropractic's Abraham Flexner: the lonely journey of John J. Nugent, 1935–1963. *Chiropractic History*, **5**, 44–57.

Haas, M., Jacobs, G.E., Raphael, R. and Petzing, K. (1995) Low back pain outcome measurement assessment in chiropractic teaching clinics: responsiveness and applicability of two functional disability questionnaires. *Journal of Manipulative and Physiological Therapies*, **18**, 79–87.

Herzog, W. and Conway, P.J. (1994) Gait analysis of sacroiliac joint patients. *Journal of Manipulative and Physiological Therapies*, **17**, 124–7.

Hildebrandt, R.W. (1967) The science of chiropractic. *ACA Journal of Chiropractic*, **4**, 58–65.

Hildebrandt, R.W. (1978) The research status of spinal manipulative therapeutics. *Journal of Manipulative Physiological Therapies*, **1**, 221–2.

Hildebrandt, R.W. (1979) Research in spinal manipulation – reflections on processes, priorities and responsibilities. *Journal of Manipulative Physiological Therapies*, **2**, 138.

Hildebrandt, R.W. (1982) Creation science and chiropractic curriculum alternatives. *Journal of Manipulative Physiological Therapies*, **5**, 53–4.

Homewood, A.E. (1979) *The Neurodynamics of the Vertebral Subluxation*, 3rd edn, Chiropractic Publishers, Toronto.

Homewood, A.E. (1988) What price research? *Dynamic Chiropractic*, 32–3.

Jamison, J.R. (1991) Science in chiropractic clinical practice: identifying a need. *Journal of Manipulative and Physiological Therapies*, **14**, 298–304.

Janse, J.J. (1976) *Principles and Practice of Chiropractic*, National College of Chiropractic, Lombard, IL.

Kawchuk, G. and Herzog, W. (1995) The reliability and accuracy of a standard method of tissue compliance assessment *Journal of Manipulative Physiological Therapies*, **18**, 298–301.

Keating, J.C., Nelson, J.M. and Mootz, R.D. (1986) A model for clinical, scientific and educational development. *Research Forum*, (Summer), 103–14.

Keating, J.C. and Calderon, L. (1987a) Clinical research preparation for chiropractors: implementing a scientist–practitioner model. *Journal of Manipulative and Physiological Therapeutics*, **10**, 124–9.

Keating, J.C. (1987b) A buddy system for chiropractic research. *Journal of the Canadian Chiropractic Association*, **31**, 9–10.

Keating, J.C. (1988) The chiropractic practitioner-scientist: an old idea revisited. *American Journal of Chiropractic Medicine*, **1**, 17–23.

Keating, J.C. (1989a) Philosophical barriers to technique research in chiropractic. *Chiropractic Technique*, **1**, 23–29.

Keating, J.C. (1989b) A survey of philosophical barriers to research in chiropractic. *Journal of the Canadian Chiropractic Association*, **33**, 184–6.

Keating, J.C. (1989c) Closing the research gap in chiropractic: a 1% solution. *Chiropractic Technique*, **1**, 62–3.

Keating, J.C. (1989d) The development of clinical research environments in the chiropractic colleges. *American Journal of Chiropractic Medicine*, **2**, 5–12.

Keating, J.C. (1989e) 50 ways to contribute to chiropractic clinical science. *Chiropractic Technique*, **1**, 109–10.

Keating, J.C. (1989f) Why shouldn't chiropractic be a first-class clinical science? *American Journal of Chiropractic Medicine*, **2**, 67–71.

Keating, J.C. (1990) Traditional barriers to standards of knowledge production in chiropractic. *Chiropractic Technique*, **2**, 78–85.

Keating, J.C. (1992) *Toward a Philosophy of the Science of Chiropractic: A Primer for Clinicians*, Stockton Foundation for Chiropractic Research, Stockton, CA.

Keating, J.C. (1993) At the crossroads: the NCA celebrates chiropractic's fortieth anniversary. *Chiropractic Technique*, **5**, 152–67.

Keating, J.C. (1995a) The age of wonderment: chiropractic in the early 20th century, in: *Chiropractic: An Illustrated History* (eds D. Peterson and G. Wiese), Mosby-Yearbook, St Louis, pp. 90 123.

Keating, J.C., Green, B.N. and Johnson, C.D. (1995b) 'Research' and 'science' in the first half of the chiropractic century. *Journal of Manipulative and Physiological Therapeutics*, **18**, 357–78.

Manga, P., Angus, D., Papadopoulos, C. and Swan, W. (1993) *The Effectiveness and Cost-Effectiveness of Chiropractic Management of Low Back Pain*, Report for the Ministry of Health, Government of Ontario, Kenilworth Publishing.

Meade, T.W., Dyer, S., Browne, W., *et al.* (1990) Low back pain of mechanical origin: randomised comparison of chiropractic and hospital outpatient treatment. *British Medical Journal*, **300**, 1431–7.

Palmer, D.D. (1910) *The Chiropractor's Adjustor: The Science, Art and Philosophy of Chiropractic*, Portland Printing House, Portland.

Peck, M.S. (1995) *In Search of Stones: A Pilgrimage of Faith, Reason, and Discovery*, Hyperion, New York, p. 299.

Rhodes, D.W., Mansfield, E.R., Bishop, P.A. and Smith, J.F. (1995a) Comparison of leg length inequality measurement methods as estimators of the femur head height difference on standing X-ray. *Journal of Manipulative and Physiological Therapies*, **18**, 448–52.

Rhodes, D.W., Mansfield, E.R., Bishop, P.A., and Smith, J.F. (1995b) The validity of the prone leg check as an estimate of standing leg length inequality measured by X-ray. *Journal of Manipulative and Physiological Therapies*, **18**, 343–6.

Shrader, T.L. (1968) A change in attitude. *ACA Journal of Chiropractic*, **5**, 21–2.

Skrabanek, P. and McCormick, J. (1989) *Follies and Fallacies in Medicine*, Tarragon Press, Glasgow.

Stude, D.E., Goertz, C. and Gallinger, M. (1994) Inter- and intraexaminer reliability of a single, digital inclinometric range of motion measurement technique in the assessment of lumbar range of motion. *Journal of Manipulative and Physiological Therapies*, **17**, 83–7.

Thorkeldsen, A. and Breen, A.C. (1994) Gray scale range and the marking of vertebral coordinates on digitized radiographic images. *Journal of Manipulative and Physiological Therapies*, **17**, 359–63.

Watkins, C.O. (1944) *The Basic Principles of Chiropractic Government*, C.O. Watkins, Sidney, MT. Reproduced as Appendix A in Keating (1992).

Watkins, C.O. (1946) Is chiropractic unity possible? *National Chiropractic Journal*, **16**(12), 29–30.

Index

Guildford College
Learning Resource Centre

Please return on or before the last date shown
This item may be renewed by telephone unless overdue

2 8 NOV 2003		
1 2 MAY 2008		

Class: _____ 615.5 VIC _____

Title: EXAMINING COMPLEMENTARY
MEDICINE
Author: _____ VICKERS, ANDREW (Ed.)